The COVID-19 Catastrophe

What's Gone Wrong and How to Stop it Happening Again

Second Edition

Richard Horton

polity

First edition published in 2020 by Polity Press
Second edition published in 2021 by Polity Press

Reprinted 2021

Polity Press
65 Bridge Street
Cambridge CB2 1UR, UK

Polity Press
101 Station Landing
Suite 300
Medford, MA 02155, USA

ISBN-13: 978-1-5095-4909-2
ISBN-13: 978-1-5095-4910-8 (pb)

A catalogue record for this book is available from the British Library.

Typeset in 12/15 Fournier MT by
Servis Filmsetting Ltd, Stockport, Cheshire
Printed and bound in the United States by LSC Communications

The publisher has used its best endeavours to ensure that the URLs for external websites referred to in this book are correct and active at the time of going to press. However, the publisher has no responsibility for the websites and can make no guarantee that a site will remain live or that the content is or will remain appropriate.

Every effort has been made to trace all copyright holders, but if any have been overlooked the publisher will be pleased to include any necessary credits in any subsequent reprint or edition.

For further information on Polity, visit our website: politybooks.com

Contents

Fear can be considered the basis for all human civilization.

Lars Svendsen, *The Philosophy of Fear* (2008)

Preface to the Second Edition

Hindsight or history? Presidents and prime ministers world-wide have argued consistently that no one could possibly have foreseen the brutal human consequences of the COVID-19 pandemic. 'Unprecedented' was, and remains, one of the most commonly used words describing this extraordinary outbreak of contagion. Those who criticise the slow early responses of many Western governments, or the complacency over prepa-rations for a second or third wave of coronavirus, or the lack of adequate support for those hit by the ensuing economic crisis, are not surprisingly censured for their apparently self-right-eous, retrospective wisdom. President Trump led the way with what one might call 'the exceptionalist defence'. In March 2020, he said, 'there's never been anything like this in history. There's never been . . . nobody's ever seen anything like this.'

It's tempting to sympathise with this point of view. The tragedy that began in December 2019, and continues still despite the allure of a vaccine, was surely unprecedented in many ways. But comforting though such a conclusion might be, it is, unfortunately, not true. And the reason is history.

Governments, scientists, doctors and citizens had a pandemic handbook readily available to guide their understanding, even their planning and decision-making. For the events that gripped our lives in 2020 can be read with uncanny and disturbing resonance in Daniel Defoe's *A Journal of the Plague Year*, published in 1722. Neither fiction nor pure documentary fact, his *Journal* described what Defoe imagined it was like to live through the Great Plague of London in 1665. His envisioning of the events of 'this calamitous year' – as they unfolded week by week, month by month – plots with devastating accuracy our own epidemic crisis today.

When the first cases of plague were reported early in 1665, London's authorities endeavoured to conceal the outbreak, echoing evidence that police officials in Wuhan, China, sought to suppress what they disingenuously called 'rumours' of a new SARS-like disease. When plague was finally accepted as a reality in London, the government was unprepared. And the public was understandably terrified as the infection took hold with forceful menace. Mental health, for example, suffered badly – a kind of 'melancholy madness' descended on England's capital.

But not everyone was affected equally. The richer elites in seventeenth-century London society were able to flee the city for the safety of their country retreats. In doing so, they left the poor behind on the frontlines of the epidemic, a frontline they faced 'with a sort of brutal courage'. The same was true for essential and mostly poorly paid workers during successive waves of COVID-19. They too bore the brunt of infection and death. Three centuries ago, London was abandoned and left desolate, just as cities across the world today have been emptied of people, confined as they have been to working from home under curfew. Music houses, theatres and shops closed in 1665. The public felt 'a kind of sadness and horror at these things'. Defoe's description is one most of us will recognise.

There was fake news in the era of plague too. 'Deceivers' proposed plague to be the judgement of an angry God. Or, insisted others, it was caused by a blazing star or comet. 'One mischief always introduces another,' wrote Defoe. The plague enabled fortune-tellers, wizards and astrologers to flourish. Quackery prospered – an array of pills, preservatives, cordials and antidotes were peddled. We should not, perhaps, have been surprised by the furore over President Trump's unevidenced advocacy of disinfectant, irradiating light and hydroxychloroquine as remedies for COVID-19.

The response by public authorities to coronavirus also mirrored that of plague – isolation and quarantine for those thought to be infected. At least we can be thankful that those living in Paris, Madrid or New York were not padlocked behind their front doors, on which was painted a bright red cross. But London's officials struggled then, just as governments around the world have done with COVID-19, to produce clear and consistent guidance for the public to follow. Physical distancing, mask wearing and ventilation were all advised then as now. Mass gatherings were prohibited. People became more conscious of their personal hygiene. Plague in the seventeenth century led to a morbid fascination with the Bills of Mortality, a statistical account of the epidemic's progress. Tormented, we too have watched the rising numbers of deaths in countries that had hitherto been able (apparently justifiably) to boast of their power, resilience and advanced healthcare – all undermined and overturned by a virus. And, just as now, in 1665 there was vigorous disagreement about the efficacy of many of these measures.

We should not be surprised that the behaviour of the public was similar across the centuries. During the first wave of lockdown in 2020, people willingly, even enthusiastically, followed the instruction to stay home. They learned to enjoy the opportunity to take up new activities. The same was true in 1665. Defoe mentions baking bread and brewing beer. Public compliance during the first wave of the 2020 pandemic successfully suppressed the outbreak. But, once it was controlled, people desperately wished to return to some level of normal life. Governments wanted to reignite their economies. Perhaps everyone was exhausted and fatigued by the 'anthropause' – this temporary cessation of humanity. The result? Many countries let their guard down and the virus bounced back – a second wave. In 1665, a similar complacency took hold. By the end of September the plague's fury was beginning to relent. People came out of their homes, shops opened, businesses resumed. The outcome of this 'imprudent rash conduct' was a second wave of plague that 'cost a great many' lives.

The economic calamity that has ensued from COVID-19 was entirely predictable. Defoe explains how manufacturing and trade were brought to 'a full stop'. He describes the 'immediate distress' that followed, rising levels of unemployment, deepening inequality, hunger and the overall 'misery of the city'. Relief provided to the poor was then through charitable assistance rather than from government furloughs and job support schemes. But the effects were similar. Here is Defoe: 'This caused the multitude of single people in London to be unprovided for; as also of families, whose living depended upon the labour of the heads of those families; I say, this reduced them to extreme misery.'

There are telling similarities between the political approaches to COVID-19 and plague too. Defoe wrote his *Journal* with a very specific purpose in mind. Plague was moving through continental Europe and was now at England's door. In 1720 in Marseilles and the surrounding region, 100,000 people died from plague – half the population. The government in England moved quickly and fearfully to protect itself. Parliament passed a Quarantine Act in 1721. The law imposed severe restrictions on individual liberty and proposed isolating whole cities or towns if they became sites of contagion. These restrictions were to be enforced 'by any kind of violence'. Violation of the law would lead to punishment by death. The Bill caused political uproar. It threatened not only to curb precious freedoms but also to interfere with commerce. A group of Tories, led by Earl Cowper, a former lord chancellor, objected and sought to have the law struck down. Defoe's *Journal* was intended to remind the public of the terrifying dangers they faced. In his view, the drastic actions that the Quarantine Act proposed were urgent and necessary – 'a public good that justified the private mischief'. In the era of COVID-19, there has been a similar resistance from libertarians to more strenuous measures to control virus transmission. Tiered controls on indoor socialising, the mixing of households, hospitality, non-essential retail, travel, and the numbers of people who could attend weddings, funerals and church services provoked fury from politicians who argued that the state's curbs on personal liberties were an affront not only to individual freedom but also to individual responsibility.

There are, of course, differences between plague and COVID-19. There were no effective therapies to treat plague. Doctors in the seventeenth century were impotent in the face of a disease for which they didn't even understand the cause. And the plague did eventually die out in December 1665, with the onset of a harsh winter. There is no expectation that our present-day coronavirus will recede into the background of our lives quite so gracefully. Mutated variants are giving the virus new life.

After twelve months, we have learned a great deal about the virus and the disease it causes. We have treatments that save lives. Over two hundred vaccine candidates are under investigation. Several have now been proven to be safe and effective. In 2021, we will see the world's largest, fastest and most coordinated effort to control a disease since the intensified smallpox eradication programme began in 1967. Indeed, smallpox provides a sobering lesson. Despite the presence of a highly effective vaccine, the last case of naturally acquired smallpox was in 1975. Today, we are not trying to eradicate a coronavirus. But it will take years, not months, before we have this pandemic under complete control. We continue to underestimate the impact of COVID-19 on our societies. One hears otherwise intelligent and sensible people talking about a return to normality by the spring or summer of 2021. But there is no simple or straightforward return to the old life that we enjoyed before COVID-19. There is only a new normal to confront.

Meanwhile, the virus continues to shock. A new variant of coronavirus – called the B.1.1.7 lineage – emerged in the UK towards the end of 2020. It is rapidly replacing other forms of the virus and is spreading well beyond Britain. Although the new variant of concern seems to be no more harmful – rates of hospitalisation and death have not, so far, increased – it is more transmissible. Scientists have estimated that the variant has a 50 to 75 per cent transmission advantage over the original 'wild type'. The R_0 of the Wuhan coronavirus was 2.5. The R_0 of B.1.1.7 lies somewhere between 2.9 and 3.2, a substantial leap in transmissibility. Although the new variant may not directly increase the number of deaths, the higher incidence of infection because of its enhanced transmissibility will indirectly increase mortality. Of special concern is the pattern of mutations in the new variant. Multiple potentially important alterations in the virus genome affect that part of the spike (S) protein binding to receptors on human cells. If sufficient numbers of mutations change the S protein in meaningful ways, the virus may be able to escape vaccine protection and evade treatments using specific antibody cocktails of the kind given to President Trump. The emergence of B.1.1.7 will not be the last surprise of this pandemic.

I wrote *The COVID-19 Catastrophe* in London during the

first period of lockdown. At that time, the worldwide mortality from the pandemic stood at 337,687 deaths. That figure has since more than quadrupled, to over 1.8 million deaths – and it continues to rise by over 10,000 deaths per day. Meanwhile, the way governments have managed the infection has had profound political consequences. To take just one example: President Trump failed to win a second term in office, despite presiding over a strong economy before the pandemic, largely because he led the worst national response to COVID-19 of any developed country in the world. The American response was characterised by chaos, division and an abundance of misinformation. A spectacular level of ineptitude enabled the country to accrue the highest number of deaths from COVID-19 of any nation – by a very long way. The political price for that failure was high and will continue to be paid for years to come.

The purpose of this second edition is not only to update figures. I have revised each chapter to try to take account of new discoveries, perspectives and interpretations. I have added an introduction that aims to reframe our understanding of COVID-19 in ways that have important consequences for protecting our communities from future pandemics. I have tried to survey some of the most difficult controversies that have emerged and what those disputes tell us about our societies. And I have added an epilogue that tries to give a provisional judgement on what the pandemic means for our future. For COVID-19 is not only a new disease caused by a new virus. It is an inflection point in our understanding about ourselves and the planet we inhabit.

Preface

COVID-19 is a pandemic of paradoxes.

Most of those who became infected with this new coronavirus suffered only mild disease, perhaps not easily shaken off, yet shaken off nevertheless. But a substantial number – perhaps as many as one in five – developed a much more severe illness, often requiring intensive care and mechanical ventilation. For far too many, COVID-19 meant that death was their destiny.

Being older and poorer and living with chronic disease were important risks for worse outcomes. Yet a significant proportion of those who endured severe illness were also young and previously fit and well.

The scientific community made an astonishing contribution to producing the new knowledge needed to guide a response to COVID-19. But many questions about the virus and the disease it causes remain unanswered, leaving important gaps in our understanding of the pandemic that make its control, even with the availability of several safe and effective vaccines, exceptionally difficult.

The World Health Organization (WHO) acted with unprecedented velocity to declare a Public Health Emergency of International Concern (PHEIC). But the world's only global health agency also struggled under intolerable political pressures to retain its credibility.

Countries pledged their support to international cooperation to defeat the pandemic. Yet those same countries were embarrassingly slow to match words with deeds, and too often they resorted to rivalry and blame.

This was a pandemic that was described and reported in terms of statistics – numbers of infections, numbers of patients in critical care and numbers of deaths. Lives were transformed into mathematical summaries. Graphs of the epidemic were drawn. And countries were compared for their rates of mortality.

But those who died cannot and should not be summarised. They must not become lines on squared paper. They must not become mere rates used to argue differences between nations. Every death counts. A person who died in Wuhan is as important as one who died in New York. Our way of describing the impact of the pandemic erased the biographies of the dead. The science and politics of COVID-19 became exercises in radical dehumanisation.

At press conference after press conference, government ministers and their medical and scientific advisors described the deaths of their neighbours as 'unfortunate'. But these were not unfortunate deaths. They were not unlucky, inappropriate or even regrettable. Every death was evidence of systematic government misconduct – reckless acts of omission that constituted breaches in the duties of public office.

I edit a medical journal, *The Lancet*, which found itself a conduit between medical scientists urgently trying to understand COVID-19 and politicians, policymakers and the public who somehow had to respond to the pandemic. As we read and published the work of these remarkable frontline workers, I was struck by the gap between the accumulating evidence of scientists and the practice of governments. As this space grew larger, I became angry. Missed opportunities and appalling misjudgements were leading to the avoidable deaths of tens of thousands of citizens. Those misjudgements were repeated during successive waves of the pandemic. There has to be a reckoning.

This book is their story.

Acknowledgements

I owe a debt of thanks to many people. To Ingrid, Isobel and Aleem, for a period of grace. To my colleagues at *The Lancet* who worked assiduously to ensure that research on COVID-19 was peer reviewed and published rapidly to support those responding on the frontlines of this pandemic. To health workers and scientists around the world who took time under immense pressure and difficulty to describe their extraordinary experiences. To John Thompson, for his constant encouragement. To Emma Longstaff, Helen Davies, Lucas Jones, Neil de Cort and Caroline Richmond from Polity, who helped to make the message real. And to three anonymous reviewers, whose comments and suggestions helped to sharpen the substance of this argument.

Introduction

'Dreadful death, fearsome with her sepulchral torch.' So wrote John Milton in his *Elegia tertia* to commemorate the death from plague of the Bishop of Winchester in 1626. The 'sepulchral torch' of the coronavirus has indeed been fearsome, causing hundreds of thousands of deaths on every continent of the world. The origin of this pandemic lay in the passage of the virus from an animal to humans – a pathological relationship between two species, with savage and deadly consequences. And yet our response to this pandemic has also yielded strangely benevolent shifts in our human–animal associations, shifts that have revealed surprising and possibly important insights into our capacities to change the world around us for the better.

The white-crowned sparrow (*Zonotrichia leucophrys*) is a common songbird in the San Francisco Bay Area. Researchers have recorded their songs over many years. They have seen that, as noise levels in city settings have risen, so songbirds have sung louder songs in order to be heard by potential territorial intruders. During the lockdown to control the first wave of the pandemic in the spring of 2020, Elizabeth Derryberry led a team of scientists intrigued by the question of whether birdsong would change when noise in the city fell sharply during its shutdown.[1]

In April and May 2020 they measured urban noise and found it had declined to levels not seen since the 1950s. They went on to record birdsong in the city and found not only that birds sang more softly during lockdown but also that, by doing so, birds could communicate over longer distances (up to twice as far) and improve their vocal performance – increasing mating potential and reducing territorial conflict. Derryberry showed how changes in human behaviour can benefit animals as well as ourselves. Songbirds rapidly recovered their vocal dexterity when noise pollution declined and the acoustic space around them was emptied. The Silent Spring of 2020 revealed that the harms human beings cause to animals can be quickly reversed. Our relationship with other species with whom we share a planet does not have to be mutually unfavourable after all.

*

It would be a mistake to call the coronavirus that causes COVID-19 'clever'. A virus is not a living, thinking, intentional creature. It is an assembly of proteins carrying a piece of genetic material – a genome – that holds the information needed to replicate itself. A virus does not breathe. It does not eat. It does not laugh. But, in its own particular way, the coronavirus that has brought our lives to a halt has qualities that are, if not admirable, then certainly deserving of our respect.

A coronavirus looks like a ball covered with spikes. Within

that ball (surrounded by a fatty or lipid membrane) is a piece – a large piece by comparison with other viruses – of genetic material called RNA, or ribonucleic acid. When viewed with a powerful electron microscope, the virus resembles a solar corona, hence its name. But don't be fooled. The spikes on the surface of the virus are not for decoration. They are the entry cards the virus uses to advance its way into human cells.

The coronavirus spikes bind to the surface of a cell (to a receptor on the membrane of the cell called ACE2, which is widely distributed in the human body). From there, the virus particle is drawn into the cell shrouded by cell membrane. The virus then releases its genome and immediately hijacks the cell's chemistry to begin the process of its own replication.

The first step in what is by now the beginning of the disease process is for the cell to 'read' particular genes contained in the viral genome. That 'translation' results in a collection of proteins that gather to form a device for reproducing thousands of copies of the viral genome. And here lies what is so exquisitely 'clever' about this coronavirus. This non-living entity has evolved a way to protect itself from genetic spelling mistakes, errors that might otherwise lead to viral extinction. The coronavirus proofreads its own work. It is able to correct errors made during the replication of the viral genome, thereby protecting its virulence and its ability to go on to harm further human cells.

Several features of this 'life cycle' of the virus make it especially difficult to destroy with a drug. First, the virus replicates itself inside a human cell. It is hard to discover a means to damage the virus while at the same time shielding the human cell. Second, a common way of disabling a virus is to block its replication by using drugs that mimic molecules essential to the replication process. But the proofreading skills the virus has evolved make the interruption of replication much more challenging. Just when you think you have introduced a catastrophic block to replication, the viral proofreader steps in to remove your intervention. And, third, the coronavirus is agile. It can change. Mutations in the genome mean that it could well evade medicines designed to target a particular piece of the genome.[2]

What we have learned about the biology of the COVID-19 coronavirus tells us that we are facing a particularly tormenting adversary.

*

What will happen to our adversary? In 2003, the first version of this coronavirus – SARS-CoV-1 – simply vanished, less than a year after it arrived. So far, it has not returned. But those coronaviruses that are more seasonal do come back, year after year, to cause variants of the common cold. Will SARS-CoV-2 disappear or will it become endemic, widely prevalent in our society, like influenza?

The answer to this question depends on the risk of reinfection. If reinfection is common, the virus will return again and again. We will live in a permanent state of vulnerability. But if reinfection is rare, it is just possible that we could drive this coronavirus out of our communities for good. Unfortunately, there have already been several reported examples of reinfection. In one case, a 25-year-old man living in Nevada tested positive on 18 April 2020, had two negative tests as part of his follow-up, but tested positive again on 5 June. Genetic analysis showed significant differences with each infection. The second infection was more severe than the first. This particular patient was infected on two separate occasions by a genetically distinct virus.[3] The alarming conclusion must be that previous exposure to the virus does not guarantee total immunity. Everyone, whether previously diagnosed with COVID-19 or not, should take identical precautions to guard against infection. But it is still too early in the pandemic to be sure how frequent reinfection will be. What we do know is that four factors will influence the risk of reinfection with this coronavirus, and so the risk of its endemicity.

The first is the degree of immunity each of us develops after infection. If immunity is long-lasting, the virus has fewer opportunities to reinfect those it infected once before. If immunity is short, reinfections will be frequent and the virus will continue to circulate in our society. The human immune response does vary in ways that might make reinfection more likely. The older one is, for example, the less effective is one's immune response. This phenomenon is called immunosenescence. Sometimes, the immune response is simply insufficient to cause immunity. Or, if it is initially sufficient, it can wane over time. The virus might also mutate, enabling it to escape whatever immunity was initially generated. (But coronaviruses mutate rather less frequently than influenza, thanks in part to their unique molecular proofreading mechanism.)

A second influence is seasonality. Is infection more common at certain times of year? For example, during the winter when people are together indoors, at school, or socially mixing in closed and crowded spaces during holidays. Strong seasonality will favour the return of the virus. Third, an interaction between viruses could play an important part in affecting reinfection. Infection with a different virus might prime the immune system, putting it on heightened alert. If a second virus arrives, one's immune system might be ready to kick into action faster than usual.

Finally, the interventions we use to lower the prevalence of the virus will shape the evolution of the pandemic. The more we adhere to good hand and respiratory hygiene and physical distancing, avoiding mass gatherings, working from home (if you can), limiting travel and wearing masks, the more we will drive the virus out of our communities. An effective drug treatment would also help, but, as I have explained, a powerful antiviral will be hard to design.

But the intervention with most potential to control this pandemic is a vaccine. The progress made towards a vaccine against COVID-19 is unrivalled. Worldwide celebrations, combined with a high dose of relief, followed in November 2020, when the pharmaceutical company Pfizer and biotechnology company BioNTech announced in a press release that their COVID-19 vaccine was more than 90 per cent effective in preventing disease. The finding, the most eagerly awaited in the recent history of public health, came from a clinical trial in over forty thousand participants. The vaccine appeared to be safe, although the trial was only just over half-complete. Dr Albert Bourla, Pfizer's chairman and chief executive, said, 'Today is a great day for science and humanity.' He was right. Until this moment, although early studies had been hopeful that a vaccine would be found, convincing evidence about the prevention of coronavirus-induced disease was not available. This achievement was indeed spectacular.

The story of the Pfizer/BioNTech vaccine was fascinating in other ways too. The founders of BioNTech were a husband and wife team – Turkish-born Chief Executive Professor Uğur Şahin and Chief Medical Officer Dr Özlem Türeci. Both are children of Turkish immigrants to Germany. Şahin was four years old when he moved to Germany and later studied medicine at the University of Cologne. Türeci grew up in a medical family – her father was a surgeon – and as a child could not imagine doing anything else but medicine. The couple met while working at the University Medical Centre in Mainz and married in 2002. Even on their wedding day, they worked in their laboratory. Together, they saw the potential of science to develop new treatments for cancer. They sold their first company, Ganymed Pharmaceuticals, in 2016 for £376 million. They created BioNTech to continue their work on cancer treatments – specifically, vaccines – based on the immune system. Until the coronavirus vaccine, none of their products had reached the bedside.

But, in January, Şahin read about the emerging pandemic in

The Lancet. Immediately, he understood the threat – and the opportunity. He moved six hundred scientists at BioNTech to begin working on a vaccine. Their approach was highly unusual. Many of the most successful vaccines – polio and measles vaccines, for example – are based on a weakened (attenuated) or inactivated form of virus. But BioNTech's vaccine uses genetic material – a type of RNA called messenger RNA, or mRNA – to stimulate immunity. The genetic sequence of SARS-CoV-2 was made publicly available by Chinese scientists on 12 January 2020. Şahin and Türeci focused on that part of the sequence which produced the spike protein on the surface of the virus. They took that sequence of mRNA, which contains the instructions to make human cells produce the spike protein, and wrapped it in a bubble of fat that enables the vaccine to enter the cell. Once inside, the mRNA uses the cell's machinery to produce large amounts of spike protein, which then sits on the surface of the cell provoking the immune response that protects that person from developing COVID-19. The vaccine enables the person who has been immunised to produce their own medicine. Many scientists had been sceptical about whether an mRNA vaccine could work. But by 11 March, when WHO officially declared COVID-19 a pandemic, BioNTech had produced twenty candidate mRNA vaccines.

During the next few months, they tested their prototype vaccines on mice, rats and monkeys and focused on four that seemed most promising. When they tested those candidates in humans, one in particular stood out as safe, as well as effective. It not only stimulated the production of antibodies to attack the virus but also triggered a parallel kind of immunity – cellular immunity – that is mediated by T cells. Their vaccine aimed to corral all the forces of the human immune system to protect the body from viral infection and disease. In July, they began the trial whose interim results were reported in November.

The UK was the first country to give regulatory approval for a vaccine – and that first vaccine was from Pfizer/BioNTech. Programmes to vaccinate priority populations began in December 2020, beginning with residents of care homes (the goal was to prioritise those at greatest risk of premature death, but it was also a poignant sign of reparation, since it was these very care home residents who had been so abandoned at the beginning of the pandemic). The US and Canada quickly followed the UK's authorisation of the Pfizer/BioNTech vaccine. Alarm was raised after only a few days of the vaccine's rollout when three recipients developed severe allergic reactions possibly linked to their immunisation. All three had a history of allergic disease. Regulators quickly revised their advice and recommended that 'any person with a history of anaphylaxis to a vaccine, medicine or food should not receive the Pfizer/ BioNTech vaccine.'

The approval of a vaccine for widespread human use was a significant milestone in the scientific response to COVID-19. Yet even this success was tinged by political controversy. The UK's minister of health, Matt Hancock, claimed that Britain had been first to approve a vaccine 'because of Brexit'. The minister of education, Gavin Williamson, went further. He said, 'I just reckon we've got the very best people in this country and we've obviously got the best medical regulator – much better than the French have, much better than the Belgians have, much better than the Americans have. That doesn't surprise me at all, because we're a much better country than every single one of them.' Although Prime Minister Boris Johnson refused to back either Hancock or Williamson, and although June Raine, chief executive of the UK's Medicines and Healthcare products Regulatory Authority, specifically refuted their claims, their nationalistic, indeed jingoistic, interpretation of the development and approval of a vaccine was a sad moment of misunderstanding. For the truth is that the science that led to the development of a vaccine against COVID-19 was the consequence of an extraordinary global collaboration – from the sequencing of the virus by Chinese scientists, to the development of the vaccine by immigrants of Turkish heritage in Germany, to its manufacture in Belgium. To be sure, the UK can be proud of its own scientists. A team led by Sarah Gilbert and Andrew Pollard at the University of Oxford had, in collaboration with AstraZeneca, developed their own vaccine against COVID-19.[4] Their vaccine received UK regulatory approval in the closing days of 2020. But the lesson of vaccine research is that the sum of scientific cooperation between nations produces greater success than can be achieved by any one group in any one country working alone.

Despite the momentous success that the discovery of a vaccine surely is, one should still be cautious. The safety profile of the vaccine will only be fully known when more people have received it and been followed for many months. Although the BioNTech vaccine prevents disease, we still don't know if those who are immunised will be able to pass on the virus. Neither do we know how long immunity will last and whether immunity will be strong in particular at-risk groups, such as older individuals. Early evidence shows that over 90 per cent of those infected with SARS-CoV-2 produce neutralising antibody responses that remain stable for several months. This finding bodes well for a sustained vaccine response. There are logistical challenges too. The vaccine has to be kept at a temperature of minus 70 to 80 degrees Celsius. Its distribution will only be possible to those places that can accommodate such stringent deep-freeze conditions. And a vaccine does not mean that we can immediately stop wearing masks or ignoring guidance on hygiene and physical distancing. There remain many unknowns.

An additional reason for optimism is that there is more than one vaccine in development. Well over two hundred vaccines are in various stages of preclinical and clinical testing. Even more importantly, different categories of vaccine are being developed. The mRNA vaccine of BioNTech is the most innovative. But three further approaches also give cause for great hope and optimism. One is the type of vaccine that uses another virus – called an adenovirus – to deliver the spike protein to the recipient's immune system. This is the type of vaccine being developed by the team in Oxford. The Gamaleya Centre in Russia and Johnson & Johnson are also at the forefront of this technology. A further approach is being led by a small US biotechnology company called Novavax. They are using moth cells to produce the spike protein, which is then attached to a soap-like particle. A purified plant compound – called a saponin – is added as an adjuvant to boost the immune response. The advantage of the Novavax vaccine is that, like the Oxford vaccine, it is stable at temperatures ranging from 2 to 8 degrees Celsius (the normal temperature of a fridge), making the logistics of its distribution much simpler. And the third approach is the most traditional – an inactivated version of the coronavirus itself.

All that said, the challenge is enormous. Most COVID-19 vaccines require two intramuscular injections. That means that, to meet full global demand, we will need at least 15 to 16 billion doses of vaccine, two doses for every person on the planet. No single pharmaceutical company will be able to deliver that amount of vaccine. The manufacturing and distribution obstacles are not trivial. It is therefore good that there is a diversity of vaccines with a wide geographic spread of development.

There is one further challenge to consider. The anti-vaccination movement is growing. Opinion polls in some countries suggest that fewer than half the eligible population would be willing to receive a coronavirus vaccine. The arguments against taking a vaccine follow a common pattern. Some claim that the dangers of the virus have been exaggerated. Others believe that the pharmaceutical industry is simply trying to profit from the pandemic. Still others argue that the speed with which vaccines are being produced surely proves that corners have been cut in safety testing. There are many websites dedicated to spreading these views through social media – for example, News Punch, Infowars and AlterNet. Elon Musk is alleged to have said that he won't allow his children to receive a COVID-19 vaccine. In the race to produce a vaccine, and in the excitement of success, far too little has been done to prepare the public for the immunisation programme that will follow. Misinformation is now a serious threat.

In their 2019 book *The Misinformation Age*, Cailin O'Connor and James Owen Weatherall explain how false beliefs persist and spread. They emphasise the social character of fake news. The connections between us in groups and networks enable the propagation of misleading evidence as well as true beliefs. Models of communication show the importance of trust in shaping the spread of beliefs. The greater the distrust among those with different views, the greater the risk of permanent polarisation. We are all also prey to conformity bias – a desire to agree with others and to trust the judgement of others. Our predilection to conformity makes it harder to take a stand against the crowd. If your network holds strong anti-vaccine views, you may find it more difficult to arrive at your own independent judgement, even if you personally are inclined to have confidence in the safety of a vaccine. And misinformation is made worse when there are active propagandists spreading fake news. Unfortunately, the field of COVID-19 vaccines is full of propagandists seeking to manipulate and mislead.

In one study by Neil Johnson and a team of American scientists, the scale of the problem facing those working to build trust in a COVID-19 vaccine was startlingly all too clear.[5] They studied 100 million people who had expressed views about vaccination and found that negative views about vaccines have become 'robust and resilient'. Anti-vaccination propagandists are relatively small numerically, but they are heavily entangled with those who are undecided about vaccine safety, giving them an opportunity to influence those who have yet to make up their mind. Pro-vaccination advocates, by contrast, tend to be more isolated from the mainstream, not only giving them fewer opportunities to influence the undecided but also leading them to believe they are winning the argument. The anti-vaxxers engage better with the undecided than do those who are pro-vaccine. Worse, although the pro-vaccine argument seems straightforward, the diverse conspiracy theories promoted by anti-vaxxers offer multiple attractive narratives to persuade the undecided. These narratives have a huge impact. The anti-vaccination movement is growing much faster than its pro-vaccination counterpart. The frightening conclusion that Johnson and his colleagues reach is that anti-vaccination views will dominate within a decade. No amount of scientific ingenuity in the development of a vaccine against COVID-19 will counter this dangerous trend.

Added to which, some COVID-19 vaccines are already in use, despite the lack of evidence from late-stage clinical trials. Russian and Chinese vaccines are being given to select populations – for example, to their armed forces in their respective countries and in the United Arab Emirates. The UAE and Bahrain have approved a vaccine developed by Chinese state-owned Sinopharm. But no data on safety or efficacy were made publicly available in advance of this decision. If one of these vaccines proves to have a serious adverse effect, and if that harm becomes headline news around the world, the damage to vaccine confidence could be irreversible.

What can be done? Although not writing about COVID-19 specifically, O'Connor and Weatherall draw conclusions that can still be applied to the present pandemic. One warning, though: they stress that anyone who thinks the 'marketplace of ideas' will sort fact from fiction is mistaken. Only an active effort to defeat misinformation will succeed.

First, social media companies, especially Facebook and Twitter, must do more to police their networks and eliminate false information about COVID-19 vaccines. If these companies do not do so, governments must intervene to force them to act. Second, trusted politicians from all political parties (and other public figures) need to speak out in support of COVID-19 vaccine science. Third, vaccine scientists must raise their standards. O'Connor and Weatherall argue that scientists should build trust by abandoning industry funding. As I have described, that isn't going to happen for a COVID-19 vaccine. Big pharma and little biotech have driven progress together towards a vaccine – a virtuous collaboration. But it is important that scientists retain maximum independence from the companies who sponsor their studies. It doesn't help to build trust when the announcement of a new vaccine result is made through a pharmaceutical company press release, as it was for the BioNTech/Pfizer vaccine. The Oxford team did better. When announcing new results, the scientists led, not corporate executives from AstraZeneca. Fourth, journalists should avoid the unwitting spread of misinformation. They must never give any kind of platform to anti-vaxxers, even in the name of 'balanced reporting'. Fifth, lawmakers can do more to regulate sources of misinformation, just as they have done for other threats to the public's health (tobacco control legislation, for example).

O'Connor and Weatherall's central claim is that 'We need to recognise fake news as a profound problem that requires accountability and investment to solve.' COVID-19 vaccine misinformation is not taken as seriously as it should be. That complacency needs to end.

*

COVID-19 is not a pandemic. The approach taken by scientists and governments worldwide to 'defeat' this coronavirus has been far too narrow. We have viewed the cause of this health emergency as the outbreak of an infectious disease. All of our interventions so far – from wearing masks to new treatments, such as the anti-viral drug remdesivir – have focused on cutting the lines of viral transmission as a means to ending the epidemic. The science that has guided governments has been driven mostly by mathematical modellers and infectious disease specialists. Understandably, they have framed the present crisis based on their knowledge of past pandemics, such as plague.

But what we have learned invites us to conclude that the story of COVID-19 is not so simple. The reality is that two categories of disease are interacting together and within specific populations: infection with a coronavirus is causing particular harm among those who are older and those who are living with chronic diseases, such as obesity, diabetes and hypertension.

Worse, these interactions are clustering within particular social groups according to patterns of inequality deeply embedded within our societies. The aggregation of these connecting conditions – viral infection and chronic non-communicable diseases – on backgrounds of social and economic disparity is worsening the adverse effects of each separate illness. COVID-19 is therefore not a pandemic. It is far worse. It is a syndemic – a synthesis of epidemics. The syndemic nature of the threat we face from COVID-19 means that a much more nuanced approach is needed if we are to protect the health of our communities.

The notion of a syndemic was first conceived in the 1990s by Merrill Singer, an American medical anthropologist. He argued that one cannot truly understand the effects of a disease by looking at that condition only in isolation. At the time, he was studying the AIDS epidemic and noticed how it was especially harming poor, urban African-American communities. He observed that HIV was often associated with other diseases, such as tuberculosis and hepatitis, all in the context of precarious social and economic conditions. These diseases and their associated risks did not simply exist side by side. Each made the other worse. AIDS worsened health outcomes if a person was poor and had additional illnesses. Equally, poverty worsened outcomes for those living with HIV. These interactions became the basis for his concept of a syndemic. His insight was to see the linkages between the biological and the social determinants of disease and to define the implications of those linkages for prognosis, treatment and broader health policies.

The conclusion for coronavirus is therefore profound. Protecting our societies from this infectious disease means paying much greater attention to the prevention and treatment of existing chronic diseases. It also means much more energetic efforts to reduce socio-economic inequalities.

Syndemics are characterised by biological and social interactions that increase a person's susceptibility to sickness or worsen their health outcomes. In the case of COVID-19, reducing or removing the predisposing effects of chronic illness will be a prerequisite for successful containment of the infection. On a global scale, the good news is that premature deaths from many chronic diseases are falling. The bad news is that the pace of that change is very slow. And for some predisposing conditions, notably obesity and diabetes, the situation is actually getting a great deal worse.

Being overweight or obese is one of the most important risk factors for a poor outcome from COVID-19. A common way of measuring weight is the body-mass index, or BMI. This index is calculated by dividing the mass of a person by the square of their height. For example, a person who weighs 75 kilograms and who is 6 feet 2 inches tall (1.88 metres) will have a BMI of 21.2 (75 divided by 1.88 squared). A BMI below 18.5 means that you are underweight. A healthy body weight lies within the range of 18.5 to 24.9. A BMI of 25 to 29.9 indicates that you are overweight; one above 30 indicates that you are officially obese.

The Global Burden of Disease is an international collaboration of over 5,000 scientists. It is based at the University of Washington in Seattle and is funded by the Bill and Melinda

Gates Foundation. Every year it produces annual estimates of mortality and morbidity for 369 diseases and 87 risk factors in 204 countries. It is the equivalent of the Human Genome Project, but for diseases rather than genes. One of the risks they track is BMI. Their findings are startling, and especially startling in the context of COVID-19. Overweight and obesity were responsible for 5 million deaths among men and women in 2019.[6] There were 56.5 million deaths that year, and so overweight and obesity contributed close to one in ten of those global deaths. That's a very high proportion.

And the problem of overweight and obesity is getting worse. In 1990, a high BMI was the ninth commonest risk causing death. By 2010, it had climbed to be the seventh commonest risk. By 2019, it was the sixth commonest risk. Between 2010 and 2019, deaths attributable to overweight and obesity rose by 32 per cent.

Protecting our communities from COVID-19 means addressing overweight and obesity, together with diabetes, hypertension, and cardiovascular and chronic respiratory diseases, among other conditions. It also means addressing the social origins of these diseases. And it means addressing the vulnerability of older citizens, especially those living in care homes; black, Asian and minority ethnic communities; and key workers who don't have the luxury of being able to work from home.

At the end of 2020, Professor Sir Michael Marmot published his prescription for tackling the social determinants of COVID-19. Although he focused on the UK, his recommendations are universally applicable. In *Build Back Fairer*, Marmot proposes much more vigorous investment in children and young people – the only way to break the chain of systemic inequality. Eliminating child poverty, spending on early years care and education, expanding and fairly rewarding the childcare workforce, establishing parenting support programmes, improving access to digital technologies, increasing training and employment opportunities for school leavers, attending to mental as well as physical health, and writing a national strategy to reduce health inequalities – these policies are indispensable for strengthening society's security against future pandemics.

The murder of George Floyd, a 46-year-old African-American man, in Minneapolis, Minnesota, on 25 May 2020, injected the issue of racial inequality into the response to COVID-19. Social and economic deprivations among ethnic minority populations have made those communities especially vulnerable to coronavirus infection and its harmful outcomes. The particularly horrific killing of George Floyd, filmed on camera for 8 minutes and 46 seconds, ignited protests worldwide and galvanised a demand for political action to address racial inequity. It also provoked doctors to insist that governments had a moral imperative to act against racism as part of their COVID-19 response.

There is a truth about COVID-19 that is barely acknowledged. No matter how effective a treatment or protective a vaccine, the pursuit of a purely biomedical solution will ultimately fail. This coronavirus has hit societies weakened by political and economic forces that have been at work over generations. The inequalities in societies that have deepened in recent years have worsened the risks from COVID-19. Unless governments devise policies and programmes to reverse these profound disparities, our societies will never be truly COVID-19 secure. We have misunderstood and underestimated what this pandemic – this syndemic – really means for each one of us.

*

The first wave of coronavirus infection in 2020 led to clear lessons that now need to be applied to successive surges of COVID-19.[7] Unfortunately, despite wide scientific consensus around these lessons, they have not been fully learned by governments.

The first lesson is that lockdowns are no permanent solution to a pandemic. When countries went into lockdown in early 2020, the public was led to believe that adhering to strict isolation would solve the approaching crisis. People complied willingly in the belief that this short, sharp shock would be a one-time event. Lockdowns succeeded in reducing viral transmission and preventing health services from becoming overwhelmed with patients suffering from COVID-19. But lockdowns on their own are not effective treatments for pandemics. Lockdowns only buy time in order to put in place other protections.

A second major lesson was that every country needs a resilient health service in order to be able to absorb the consequences of an outbreak as severe as COVID-19. Resilience means having adequate supplies of personal protective equipment and sufficient hospital high-dependency and intensive-care facilities, including ventilators, and qualified health professionals to deliver that care. Only by embedding this additional capacity within the health system can one prevent the cancellation of non-emergency care services, which happened in many European countries. The health system also needs to be able to incorporate social care within its planning. The discharge of patients with COVID-19 from hospitals into care homes without testing, with the result that many older care-home residents became infected, was at least partly because the health and social care systems operated independently of each other.

Third, countries need robust public health systems. Two aspects of public health proved critical to success – leadership and an effective test, trace and isolate system. Countries that performed well during the first wave of the pandemic had clear and effective leadership in translating evidence into policy, often with national public health institutions playing a key part (the Robert Koch Institute in Germany was a good example). When public health institutions were sidelined, as took place in the US, where President Trump ignored advice from the respected Centers for Disease Control and Prevention, the transfer of reliable knowledge to decision-makers was hampered. The lack of adequate test, trace and isolate systems was an additional serious weakness for many countries. The absence of testing systems that could deliver results within 24 hours or the lack of teams of tracers who could follow up contacts meant that countries were frequently ill-prepared for a second wave of infection. South Korea performed well during the first wave of the pandemic partly because its test, trace and isolate system was logistically better prepared than those in many other countries. (South Korea also benefited from high levels of trust in its government, which contributed to high levels of compliance with isolation. Not all countries have been so fortunate in preserving trust in government authorities.)

There are different views about how aggressive a test, trace and isolate system should be. When levels of virus in the community are high, any testing and tracing system is going to be challenged. The number of contacts would simply overwhelm tracing capacity. But when community transmission has been controlled – e.g., in the immediate aftermath of a lockdown – a well-organised testing and tracing system has an important part to play in reducing opportunities for further viral spread, providing there is a high compliance with self-isolation.

Perhaps the most ambitious proposal for testing came from Julian Peto, an epidemiologist at the UK's London School of Hygiene and Tropical Medicine. His idea is universal repeated testing – testing the whole population weekly and insisting on strict quarantine if a test is positive. Quarantine would end when all members of a household tested negative. All infected and potentially infected individuals will be removed from the possibility of further transmitting the virus, thereby enabling the rest of society to continue to live normally (but still complying with measures such as hand and respiratory hygiene, mask wearing and physical distancing). But unfortunately, as we have seen in many Western countries, governments and public health systems have struggled to get even a minimally effective test, trace and isolate system up and running.

A fourth lesson was the importance of building trust between the public and government through clear communication and support. The importance of trust and communication was underestimated by political leaders in many countries. Disputes over physical distancing, mask wearing, the closure of schools and universities, the advisability of going to work (or not), and attendance at mass gatherings became sources of friction in many nations. The lack of consistency in advice to the public was often understandable. It took some time for scientists to understand, for example, that a coronavirus could be transmitted in aerosol form – that is, it could hang in small particles in the air and not fall immediately under the force of gravity onto surfaces. But these disagreements took their toll. Commentators sometimes took campaigning positions against the scientific mainstream. One example in the UK was Peter Hitchens. He persistently criticised the government for its advice to wear masks. Hitchens called masks 'face nappies' and 'face muzzles', claiming that the public was being turned into voiceless submissives.

A final lesson concerns national borders. The World Health Organization has consistently recommended against travel or trade restrictions to countries experiencing COVID-19 outbreaks. Their arguments are persuasive. Spending time trying to police a closed border might take precious resources, especially people, away from other more effective interventions. Travel restrictions might also interrupt aid and technical support. Or they could worsen the adverse economic impacts on a country. But early in a pandemic, or as a country is exiting lockdown, having open borders does renew the risk of importation of new infections. Several Asian countries (Japan, South Korea, Singapore, Hong Kong) implemented strict border controls as part of their pandemic response, often with mandatory testing and fourteen-day quarantine to cover the full incubation period of the virus.

There are two footnotes to these lessons. One is that government authorities must have accurate data in order to make effective decisions. For high-income countries, despite the difficulties over test and trace systems, offices of national statistics are usually able to provide highly reliable information to governments. But for many low-income countries health information systems are commonly weak or even non-existent. If a pandemic hits, governments will be flying blind. They will not have the people, equipment or resources to investigate an outbreak of a new infectious disease. For many countries in sub-Saharan Africa and South Asia, this lack of reliable information has been their most severe challenge.

A second footnote is that science made a huge contribution to the response to COVID-19 by providing evidence to guide politicians. Having a well-funded research system – universities, research institutes, laboratories and a high-quality scientific workforce – didn't guarantee success (just look at the response of the US and the UK). But science – specifically, a more open, transparent, collaborative and socially engaged science – certainly helped the public to understand the threat of this new coronavirus and enabled the rapid development of new treatments and vaccines. As economies struggle during the next five years to return to growth, there will be a temptation to trim public expenditure. There will be many competing claims on the public purse. I hope that as ministers of finance review spending they will remember that a strong research system is as much about homeland and economic security as it is about discovery and knowledge.

*

There was another lesson too. And it was one that may not have been anticipated. In 2019, *The Lancet* published a study from the Council of Foreign Relations, based in Washington, DC. Thomas Bollyky and his colleagues investigated the relation between democracy and health.[8] They correlated a country's regime type with measures of life expectancy and mortality and found that 'democracies are more likely than autocracies to lead to health gains.' Before COVID-19, we might have agreed with that view – the intrinsic advantages that democracies have over other types of political system. No longer.

The worst outcomes of COVID-19 – measured by deaths per 100,000 of the population – were to be found in democratic nations. The ten countries that have the worst mortality outcomes, at the time of writing, are Belgium, Peru, Spain, Italy, the UK, Argentina, Mexico, Bosnia and Herzegovina, the US and Brazil. Belgium ranks 33 out of 167 countries in *The Economist*'s annual Democracy Index (from 2019). In descending order, the democracy rankings for the poorest performing coronavirus countries after Belgium are 58, 16, 35, 14, 48, 73, 102, 25 and 52. Nine of these ten countries are concentrated in the top half of democracies in the world. Bosnia and Herzegovina is an outlier. Why did some of the worst outcomes arise in what we would judge to be some of the more politically advanced and pluralist societies in the world?

Does the answer lie in the degree of political populism in a country? There seems to be some relationship. President Trump, Prime Minister Boris Johnson, President Jair Bolsonaro and President Andrés Manuel López Obrador are all populists, in the sense that they have defined themselves as the champions of ordinary citizens. But the governments of Belgium, Spain and Italy are certainly not populist. And some of the most populist countries in, for example, Europe performed well. Viktor Orbán is the avowedly populist prime minister of Hungary. But he has presided over a COVID-19 mortality rate of 19 per 100,000. The figures for the UK, Spain and Italy are 81, 91 and 79, respectively.

The likely answer, in truth, is that there is no single explanation for why democracies performed poorly when compared with more authoritarian political regimes. But one factor I think we can say contributed to higher death rates – a loss of public trust in government, a loss that was exacerbated when pluralistic debate mutated into political sectarianism.

The name of Dominic Cummings has attracted wider importance than the impact of his work as chief political advisor to Prime Minister Boris Johnson probably deserves. But his name will go down in COVID-19 history nevertheless. On 22 May, *The Guardian* and the *Daily Mirror* reported that Cummings had broken lockdown rules by driving 420 km with his wife and child to a second family home. When challenged about his actions, Cummings neither apologised nor resigned. Instead, he denied any wrongdoing in an extraordinary televised address from the Downing Street Rose Garden. Johnson fully backed his political advisor. But Daisy Fancourt and a team from the Department of Behavioural Science and Health at University College London showed that these events badly damaged confidence in the government's ability to manage the pandemic.[9] By examining measures of public confidence, they showed that, starting on 22 May, there was an abrupt fall in confidence in England, a decrease that continued over the next few days and which didn't recover. There was no evidence of similar losses of confidence in the Scottish or Welsh governments, indicating this was a specific Cummings effect on the government of which he was a part. Confidence in Johnson's government has continued to remain low.

Trust also began to break down in other, even more insidious, ways. A breach in politicians' and the public's faith in science began to emerge. As countries faced a resurgence of coronavirus transmission towards the end of August, scientific advisors began to recommend further mandates and restrictions. But whereas in March people were ready to stay at home to protect their health and to prevent their health services from becoming overwhelmed, the growing economic emergency started to generate resistance to the scientists and their message. And those scientists began to be targets for public opprobrium. 'Britain is in the grip of mad science', wrote one political commentator in October. 'Boris is now a prisoner of the scientists', ran a newspaper headline. Robert Dingwall, a professor of sociology, commented that 'we have found ourselves in the hands of a scientific and medical elite with limited understanding of humanity and its needs.'

The reasons for this crisis in the science of COVID-19 were mostly self-inflicted. An early consensus about how to manage the spread of the virus disintegrated. Scientists splintered into factions. In the UK, division began with the creation of an independent Scientific Advisory Group for Emergencies, chaired by Sir David King, a former chief scientific advisor to the government. The rupture continued with increasingly personal attacks. Oxford University's Carl Heneghan and Tom Jefferson wrote in the *Mail on Sunday*: 'It is unfortunate that Mr Johnson is surrounded by mediocre scientific advisors.' Heneghan, Jefferson and others developed their opposition in an open letter arguing that the UK government's policies, based on advice from its chief medical officer and chief scientific advisor, were causing 'significant harm across all age groups'. Other scientists organised a counter-letter expressing strong support for a policy 'to suppress the virus across the entire population.' Dingwall suggested this view was simply an example of scientists' self-interest – 'Laboratory scientists . . . need to justify their research funding', he wrote. The media interpreted these fractures as indicating severe dysfunction in the relation between science and government. 'How can we follow the science when scientists haven't the foggiest?', concluded one observer.

And it seemed that some scientists advising government were cashing in on a national emergency by having substantial financial interests in businesses engaged in COVID-19 work. One newspaper headline drew striking attention to these alleged conflicts of interest: 'Government test tsar has £770k shares in firm that sold us £13m of "pointless" kits.'

What are politicians and the public to make of these divisions and allegations? They are likely to be perplexed. And that perplexity could easily and quickly, as it did with Dominic Cummings, turn into mistrust. One corrosive feature of the pandemic was that, as it proceeded, scientists were no longer seen as providing impartial, independent advice to government. They were instead blamed for crashing economies, driving up unemployment, and ruining livelihoods. They were accused of leaking sensitive documents to journalists, promoting their own personal beliefs, and collaborating with opposition political parties. Science has made a hugely positive contribution to understanding and managing the coronavirus pandemic. But COVID-19 has also provided a platform for some scientists and journalists recklessly to exploit a crisis that threw up inevitable uncertainties and contingencies.

*

Lockdowns became the quintessential symbol of COVID-19. Shutting down society was the only tool governments had that could guarantee turning off viral transmission – instructions to stay at home; restrictions on travel; closing schools and universities; mandates to stop socialising; shutting hospitality and entertainment venues, non-essential shops, close contact services (such as hairdressers) and sports facilities and gyms; limiting numbers of people attending weddings and funerals; and curfews. These measures, together with rules on hygiene, physical distancing, shielding of the sick and those aged over seventy, self-isolation if symptomatic, and mask wearing, were called 'non-pharmaceutical interventions'. The combined effect of these actions was consistently shown to be the only way to push the reproduction number, R, below 1. Indeed, modelling studies by scientists at the London School of Hygiene and Tropical Medicine showed not only that these extreme measures were required to bring the epidemic under control, but also that these intensive interventions with periodic lockdown periods would need to be in place permanently until either herd immunity was achieved through repeated waves of infection or a vaccine became available.

But lockdowns come with a terrible human cost. In England, for example, lockdowns reduced the number of patients with acute heart disease admitted to hospital. The fall in admissions showed the success of stay-at-home orders. But this reduced number of acutely ill people admitted to hospital resulted in increases in deaths from heart disease out of hospital. In France, the same pattern was observed. Worse, French scientists reported that cardiac arrests outside hospital doubled during lockdown, presumably because those who developed symptoms of chest pain stayed away from hospital.

A similar effect was seen for those with cancer. For countries implementing lockdowns, the expectation is that diagnostic delays will lead to a sharp increase in deaths over the next five years for those with cancers of the breast, colon and lung. Indeed, when lockdowns were lifted, health services faced a large backlog of patients with undiagnosed later stage cancer. Mental health was a further casualty of lockdowns. In the UK during the first lockdown, clinically significant levels of mental distress rose. The effects were particularly harsh for young people between the ages of eighteen and thirty-four, women, and people living with young children. General practice saw a halving of diagnoses of common mental health conditions, such as anxiety disorders and depression, during lockdown. Again, lockdowns appear to leave a large number of patients uncared for and with undiagnosed illness. The UK's Royal College of Psychiatrists has predicted that COVID-19 poses the greatest threat to mental health since the Second World War.

In less well-resourced countries, the impacts of lockdown went even further. In Nepal, for example, births taking place in hospital plummeted by 50 per cent. The result was a tragic and preventable increase in stillbirths and neonatal deaths. Lockdowns severely diminished the quality of care during pregnancy and childbirth. And in Bangladesh women reported reductions in paid work, increases in extreme poverty, rising levels of food insecurity, worsening depression and anxiety, and increased physical and emotional violence.

It was therefore entirely reasonable for politicians and the public to ask, when the second wave of the pandemic came, whether there was another way. Lockdowns are brutal, blunt instruments of national coercion. A group of infectious disease epidemiologists and public health scientists came together to offer an alternative to lockdown. They issued what they called the Great Barrington Declaration, named after the town in Massachusetts where the American Institute for Economic Research (which provided assistance pro bono) is located. The Declaration was written in October 2020 by Dr Jay Bhattacharya (a professor of medicine at Stanford University), Dr Sunetra Gupta (an infectious disease specialist at the University of Oxford) and Dr Martin Kulldorff (a biostatistician at Harvard University). Its purpose was to address 'how the current COVID-19 strategies are forcing our children, the working class, and the poor to carry the heaviest burden.' In place of lockdowns, the Declaration recommended 'focused protection'. Its authors explain:

> The most compassionate approach that balances the risks and benefits of reaching herd immunity is to allow those who are at minimal risk of death to live their lives normally to build up immunity to the virus through natural infection, while better protecting those who are at highest risk. We call this Focused Protection.

The response was swift. A counter-movement of scientists with interests ranging from infectious disease to paediatrics, from health policy to epidemiology, collaborated to write what they termed the John Snow Memorandum, named after the man who, in 1854, famously removed the handle of a water pump on Broad Street in London, thereby ending an outbreak of cholera and proving that the disease was transmitted by water. They called focused protection 'a dangerous fallacy'. They wrote:

> Any pandemic management strategy relying upon immunity from natural infections for COVID-19 is flawed. Uncontrolled transmission in younger people risks significant morbidity and mortality across the whole population. In addition to the human cost, this would impact the workforce as a whole and overwhelm the ability of healthcare systems to provide acute and routine care.

But this debate presented a false choice. The attractive deceit was that individual responsibility was the way out of this predicament. In the UK, a group of Conservative Party members of the House of Lords, led by the science writer (Viscount) Matt Ridley, wrote in *The Times* in October that 'Anyone who wishes to resume normal life, and take the risk of catching the virus, should be free to do so.' But while opinions might vary, the facts of the second wave were indisputable. In all European countries, and across North America, the incidence of COVID-19 was increasing in all age groups. A generalised epidemic was emerging. The R value was above 1 in most locations. Infections were doubling every seven to fourteen days. Systems of testing, tracing and isolating those in contact with infection were not working well. Study after study showed that over 90 per cent of the population was still susceptible to infection after the first wave. And the burden of COVID-19 was still falling on the frailest and most vulnerable in society. This disease cannot be solved through individual responsibility alone. The state is responsible for the health of its citizens. It is therefore government that must intervene to protect the public's health and wellbeing. Tiered mandates reduce infections, hospitalisations and deaths. They buy time to put in place additional public health protections. And the lesson of the initial lockdown is that the best time for a precautionary break is always yesterday.

*

An epidemic of acute infection gave way to an epidemic of chronic illness – known as 'Long COVID'. It's still too early to be sure what the long-term consequences of COVID-19 will be. Only studies lasting over the next few years and decades will give us answers. But what we do know is that SARS-CoV-2 causes a wide array of symptoms and syndromes in a large proportion of those infected for three to six months after they have recovered from COVID-19 – perhaps as many as three-quarters of patients. The most commonly described symptoms are fatigue, muscle weakness and sleep difficulties. Almost half of those infected have continuing difficulties with smell. A quarter go on to report anxiety and depression. COVID-19 usually begins as a pneumonia, and so it is not surprising that long-term lung damage is common, especially in those who suffered the most severe forms of disease. But there is also a long list of reported health problems – among them, headache, tremors, walking difficulties and cognitive deficits. A third of those who recovered endured a worse quality of life. One in ten suffered post-traumatic stress disorder. Importantly, post-COVID-19 illness was more common among women.

The evidence so far suggests that Long COVID may not be a single condition. The spike protein on the surface of the coronavirus binds to a receptor on the surface of human cells called ACE2 (the angiotensin-converting enzyme 2 receptor). This receptor is found in the lungs, heart, gastrointestinal tract, kidneys, blood vessels and nervous system. With such a wide variety of organs susceptible to attack by the virus, it is not surprising that the short-term and long-term presentations of illnesses associated with SARS-CoV-2 are also so varied. Four distinct groups of symptoms seem to exist under the diagnostic umbrella of Long COVID. First, brain fog, a kind of interruption of normal thought. Second, shortness of breath, linked to long-term damage to the lungs. Third, abnormalities of cardiac rhythm, caused by the direct effects of the virus on the heart. And, fourth, high blood pressure, probably because the virus also targets blood vessels. The lesson of Long COVID is that this coronavirus should not be underestimated. The introduction of a vaccine will prevent Long COVID from growing in size. But, with over 80 million confirmed cases of COVID-19 already reported, the potential for huge present and future suffering is great.

One distinctive observation about COVID-19 is the steep age gradient among those who develop severe disease. About half of those who die of COVID-19 are over the age of eighty. A third are between the ages of sixty and seventy-nine. That means over 90 per cent of deaths are among those over sixty; 8

per cent are aged between forty and fifty-nine, while less than 1 per cent of deaths are of people below the age of forty. The fact that COVID-19 is not a young person's disease means that the effects of the pandemic on children and young people have been largely overlooked.

But children have suffered (and are suffering) significant harm to their health from COVID-19. These harms could well cause long-term damage to a whole generation – increased levels of poverty, disrupted vaccination programmes causing the re-emergence of vaccine-preventable diseases (such as measles), higher newborn and child mortality because of health services thrown into disarray, worsened mental health (including increased numbers of suicides), increased rates of child marriage, and violence in the home under lockdown. Girls are especially at risk from dropping out of school as families re-enter poverty.

Children do get infected with this coronavirus. Some develop symptoms of fever, a dry cough, and even pneumonia. But, thankfully, most children develop only mild or moderate COVID-19. Many children, perhaps a third, suffer no symptoms at all (a dangerous fact for those trying to reduce community-acquired infections). COVID-19 is highly transmissible, similar to influenza, but can have a covert presentation in children. Children who do become infected are young, with an average age of five years, and a small proportion go on to develop a more severe form of COVID-19, requiring admission to intensive care and prolonged ventilation. A fatal outcome is exceedingly unusual. Therefore, the good news for children is that the coronavirus seems to cause a much milder immunological response with less immune damage. SARS-CoV-2 is much more merciful in children than in adults. The reasons why remain unclear.

During the initial lockdown over 1 billion children – over 90 per cent of the world's student population – stopped attending school. This withdrawal from educational settings for two months or more is far more likely to have affected children adversely than becoming infected with the virus itself. It also reduced parent and carer participation in work, with severe consequences for staff shortages in essential services, such as healthcare. And yet as the evidence was gathered it became clear that schools were not the COVID-19 hot spots once thought. Studies of schools showed that the number of cases of COVID-19 was low. As the pandemic evolved, mounting evidence indicated that the closure of schools had been an unnecessary, if understandable, overreaction, one that will have deepened inequalities and harmed the very poorest children and young people in society. A survey of schools during the pandemic by *Science* magazine revealed that most schools in India, Indonesia and Mexico remained shut. 'The inequities from school to school are inexcusable and heart-wrenching', reported one headmaster. Schools that did continue to operate during the first wave did not contribute significantly to the spread of infection. The lesson is that, provided other measures are in place (enhanced hygiene, physical distancing, ventilation, appropriate mask wearing, and testing), schools can remain open in a safe way for the educational, social and economic good of the community as we adapt to living with COVID-19. Even with the emergence of new and more transmissible variants of coronavirus, the decision to keep schools open is not a scientific question. It is a moral and political necessity.

Universities are a more complicated story. They have been hit hard by the pandemic. In the UK, for example, more than 3,000 staff were made redundant in 2020. Universities face a financial as well as an educational crisis. When students returned to college campuses in September 2020, infections surged. No health crisis ensued because young people are at a far lower risk of serious disease. Yet those students may still be a danger, if not to themselves, then to those living in surrounding local communities. There is evidence that rates of death in college communities have been higher than elsewhere. And genetic fingerprinting indicates that these deaths are connected to outbreaks in universities. Some health officials have criticised students for failing to adhere rigorously to the rules of self-isolation if infected. But it would be unfair to single out students for special condemnation. The truth is that, after a year of disruption, many of us may have stretched the boundaries of our behaviour. We may have redefined the limitations of mandates. And we may have justified our choices in the face of fatigue and frustration. Students and their universities were simply a microcosm of the rest of society.

But these mostly reassuring messages were tempered by the discovery of a surprising, rapidly emerging, severe and rare new disease in a small proportion of children who became infected with SARS-CoV-2. As the pandemic swept through

Italy, paediatricians noticed that children with COVID-19 developed a condition similar to Kawasaki disease. This disease is an acute and usually self-limiting inflammation of the blood vessels (a vasculitis), especially coronary arteries, which almost exclusively affects previously healthy young infants and children. The cause of Kawasaki disease, which was first reported by Tomisaku Kawasaki in Tokyo in 1961, is unknown but is thought to be related to an infectious agent. The Italian paediatricians found that the incidence of Kawasaki disease increased thirtyfold during the first wave of the pandemic. Children presented with fever, shock, abdominal pain, vomiting and diarrhoea. They had a higher incidence of severe forms of the disease that especially affected the heart. They were older and often showed damage to the lungs and digestive tract. A small number of these children died. Other countries began to see the same pattern of multisystem inflammatory symptoms in children, symptoms severe enough to require admission to intensive care and ventilation. The current view is that this Kawasaki-like disease is distinct from that originally described by Tomisaku Kawasaki. Children with similar presentations are older and have a more intense inflammatory response. As a result, it seems that COVID-19 has unleashed a new disease among children – paediatric inflammatory multisystem syndrome temporally associated with SARS-CoV-2, or PIMS-TS.

Relative to their risk of contracting disease, children have been disproportionately affected by the COVID-19 pandemic, and especially by lockdowns. The impact on education in 2020 may adversely affect an entire generation. COVID-19 threatens to reverse twenty-five years of progress in child health.

Where will the era of COVID-19 lead us? In 1960, the French sociologist Raymond Aron delivered a lecture in London entitled 'The Dawn of Universal History'. He argued that countries were converging towards one and the same history – a history in which all humankind had access to the same tools. The spread of this industrial society meant, Aron claimed, that the world was moving from a time characterised by division to one defined by unification – 'the beginning of a united mankind engaged in the only worthwhile struggle, the one for mastery over nature and the wellbeing of all humanity.' His optimism was premature. The past sixty years have seen neither the diminution of conflict nor the erasure of ideology. But perhaps COVID-19, an acute global phenomenon, will usher in a single universal history. Not the end of history, but the beginning of a new history – one in which humanity will join and act together for the interests of all in the name of all. A dreamy and quixotic imagining? No, I think necessary and inevitable.

From Wuhan to the World

> While the human race battles itself, fighting over ever more crowded turf and scarcer resources, the advantage moves to the microbes' court. They are our predators and they will be victorious if we, *Homo sapiens*, do not learn how to live in a rational global village that affords the microbes few opportunities.
>
> It's either that or we brace ourselves for the coming plague.
>
> Laurie Garrett, *The Coming Plague* (1994)

Something happened. The precise details still remain uncertain and may never be fully uncovered. But here is what one can reasonably be sure of so far.

On 30 December 2019, samples were taken from the lungs of a patient with a mysterious pneumonia. He had been admitted to Wuhan Jin Yin-tan Hospital in Wuhan, Hubei Province, China. A test called real-time reverse transcriptase polymerase chain reaction (RT-PCR) confirmed the presence of a new type of coronavirus.

Coronaviruses are common in animals, such as bats, cats and camels. There are hundreds of different types of coronavirus. Six had been known to infect human beings – spillover infections into humans from their animal hosts. They are responsible for around 10 to 15 per cent of cases of the common cold.

Four human coronaviruses cause only mild to moderate symptoms – NL63 (identified in the Netherlands in 2004), HKU1 (discovered in Hong Kong in 2005) and OC43 and 229E (both major causes of the common cold). But two coronaviruses pose much more serious threats to human health – Severe Acute Respiratory Syndrome coronavirus (SARS-CoV-1) and Middle-East Respiratory Syndrome coronavirus (MERS-CoV). Could the virus discovered in Wuhan be a seventh and also more dangerous type of coronavirus?

The genetic code of the novel virus was quickly sequenced by Chinese scientists. Comparisons with existing viral genomes showed that it was closely related to a bat SARS-like strain. Those four letters – S-A-R-S – struck fear and not a little panic into Chinese health officials when the news arrived in Beijing. An outbreak of SARS in 2002–3 had infected 8,096 people and caused 774 deaths across 37 countries (a disturbingly high 10 per cent mortality rate). The political mishandling of that epidemic had brought widespread international criticism of China's leaders. A repeat of that national humiliation could not be allowed.

The early response to the discovery of this new SARS-like virus, eventually named SARS-CoV-2, was one of paralysing anxiety. Li Wenliang was working as an ophthalmologist in Wuhan. On 30 December, he privately alerted medical friends and colleagues through his WeChat account about the existence of the new SARS virus. When his online posts leaked and reached the local Wuhan police, he was detained, questioned and admonished for 'rumour-mongering'. Li was forced to sign a statement confirming that he would stop spreading these alleged rumours. Local Communist Party officials in China like to keep a low profile with Beijing. Post-Tiananmen, their primary duty is to preserve public order and stability. In their eyes, Li Wenliang had to be gagged.

Meanwhile, a health alert was released by Wuhan's local government authorities on 31 December. Doctors in Wuhan had noticed that several patients admitted to hospital with this new virus-like disease shared a common story – they had all visited Huanan seafood market, a live-animal and seafood wholesale market in the city. The source of the original SARS outbreak in 2002–3 was eventually traced to civets, cat-like mammals that resemble ferrets, which had in turn become infected from bats. Was the same sequence of events now repeating itself? Had the new SARS-like virus again jumped from animals to humans (this type of species transfer is called a zoonotic infection)? It seemed likely. The market was shut down on 1 January.

The Chinese government had learned lessons from 2002–3. As soon as Beijing officials confirmed the report from Wuhan, they posted news of the outbreak on the website of the Wuhan Municipal Health Commission. WHO's Country Office in Beijing picked up this media statement, translated it, and notified its Western Pacific Regional Office in Manila. WHO also noted a media report from an organisation called ProMED about the same cluster of cases in Wuhan. On 1 January, WHO set up an Incident Management Support Team to investigate the outbreak and requested further information from the Chinese government about the outbreak. On 2 January, WHO began to spread word about the outbreak by informing the Global Outbreak Alert and Response Network partners about the new infectious threat. By 3 January, forty-four cases of the new disease had been reported. Worryingly, these patients were not suffering from the common cold. Eleven had very severe pneumonia. Chinese officials now began to work with WHO on this 'viral pneumonia of unknown cause'.

The next day, WHO alerted the world to this outbreak via Twitter: 'China has reported to WHO a cluster of pneumonia cases – with no deaths – in Wuhan, Hubei Province. Investigations are underway to identify the cause of this illness.' On 5 January, the agency made a more formal official notification of the outbreak, and on 10 January it issued technical guidance about how to detect, test and manage new cases of the disease.

Twenty years after the first outbreak of SARS, Chinese science was far better prepared. The country's scientists quickly isolated the virus and sequenced its genome, which they shared publicly on 12 January.

The next day, the first case of infection outside China was reported – WHO issued a statement saying that a traveller from Wuhan had arrived in Thailand and had been hospitalised on 8 January. It emphasised that 'The possibility of cases being identified in other countries was not unexpected, and reinforces why WHO calls for ongoing active monitoring and preparedness in other countries.'

Dr Tedros Adhanom Ghebreyesus, WHO's director-general, now realised he had the makings of a health crisis on his hands. His predecessor, Dr Margaret Chan, had been criticised for being slow to respond to the outbreak of Ebola virus in West Africa, which began in December 2013. That outbreak led to over 11,000 reported deaths. Like China over SARS, WHO could not afford to be seen to fail again. The agency said that Dr Tedros 'will consult with Emergency Committee members and could call for a meeting of the committee on short notice.'

The committee in question was the International Health Regulations (IHR) Emergency Committee. The IHR are legally binding rules designed 'to prevent, protect against, control, and provide a public health response to the international spread of disease.' If a disease endangers international public health, the committee can recommend, and the director-general of WHO can issue, a Public Health Emergency of International Concern (PHEIC).

The declaration of a PHEIC is, in the words of the IHR, 'an extraordinary event'. It is probably the most extraordinary power that a director-general of WHO possesses. Although they must consult a country about a disease threat, they are free to ignore their views or wishes. It is the decision of the director-general alone as to whether there is enough evidence for a PHEIC to be issued. This is serious power.

Ebola was first reported in Guinea in December 2013, before spreading to Liberia and Sierra Leone. The case fatality was 40 per cent. Individuals with Ebola virus disease were identified in Mali and Nigeria. The infection was also transported to the US, the UK, Italy and Spain. Dr Chan declared a PHEIC on 8 August 2014, eight months after the first cases of Ebola were described. The need to avoid a similar delay would have weighed heavily on the mind of Dr Tedros. He needed to evaluate the available evidence about what was happening in Wuhan carefully, but also quickly.

There are two criteria that must be met for a PHEIC to be declared. First, the disease must constitute a public health risk to other states through the international spread of that disease. Second, the disease must potentially require a coordinated international response in order to control it.

At the first Emergency Committee meeting on 22–3 January 2020, members were evenly split as to whether they should recommend a PHEIC. Many informed observers were surprised. When the threat of a new infectious disease emerges, the common view, based on past failures, is that one should have a very low threshold for calling a global red alert. But Dr Tedros paused. Without the backing of the Emergency Committee he wasn't prepared to act alone. He needed more evidence – and time.

His anxieties only worsened when, on 24 January, a team of Hong Kong scientists published findings in *The Lancet* showing that the novel coronavirus could be transmitted from person to person. Ominously, they directly compared the new outbreak with the 2002–3 SARS epidemic, and they made several important recommendations:

Learning from the SARS outbreak, which started as animal-to-human transmission during the first phase of the epidemic, all game meat trades should be optimally regulated to terminate this portal of transmission. But . . . it is still crucial to isolate patients and trace and quarantine contacts as early as possible because symptomatic infection appears possible . . ., educate the public on both food and personal hygiene, and alert health-care workers on compliance to infection control.[1]

While scientists were dissecting the genetics and biology of the virus, doctors were struggling to manage the disease it caused. This condition was no straightforward pneumonia. Although many patients who contracted the infection had a mild illness and recovered quickly, a large subgroup (around 20 per cent) developed a much more severe form of the disease. Common presenting symptoms were fever, cough, muscle pain and fatigue. But if you were male, older and had a pre-existing disease, such as diabetes, high blood pressure, obesity or a heart condition, you seemed more likely to become critically ill – and die.

The onset of severe illness was usually heralded by shortness of breath about a week after the initial symptoms. There then ensued a rapid progression to acute respiratory distress syndrome, requiring mechanical ventilation on an intensive-care unit (ICU). And then a pathological explosion took place. A storm of chemicals called cytokines was unleashed on the body. Patients developed multiple organ failures – acute injuries of the heart, kidneys and liver, blood clots in small vessels, and secondary infections. All doctors could do was mechanically ventilate and support patients on ICU as best they could and hope they pulled through. Half of those admitted to ICU didn't.

The first clinical description of the disease, which would later be called COVID-19, was also published on 24 January.[2] The authors of that report were clearly alarmed by what they were seeing. They described a 'serious, sometimes fatal, pneumonia' that 'required ICU admission'. They reported that 'The number of deaths is rising quickly' and noted that 'Airborne precautions, such as a fit-tested N95 respirator, and other personal protective equipment are strongly recommended.' They underlined the fact that COVID-19 shared 'some resemblance to SARS-CoV and MERS-CoV infections'. They emphasised that no treatment existed. And they stressed 'the pandemic potential' of the new coronavirus. The story of the next twelve months was described in that single paper.

Dr Tedros visited China and met President Xi Jinping on 28 January. He was beginning to understand the enormous gravity of the outbreak, and on 30 January he reconvened the IHR Emergency Committee. This time there was no split. The committee recommended action. Dr Tedros declared a PHEIC the same day. In WHO's own words, a PHEIC 'implies a situation that: is serious, unusual, or unexpected; carries implications for public health beyond the affected State's national border; and may require immediate international action.'

It had taken thirty days, not eight months, to issue WHO's highest category of international alert. The world had been warned. And it was still only January.

The 'pandemic potential' of SARS-CoV-2 was further

highlighted by Gabriel Leung and a team of scientists at the University of Hong Kong on 31 January. They too understood the danger the world faced. As the capital city of Hubei Province, Wuhan is a major domestic and international transport hub. Flights out of Wuhan carried passengers to Bangkok, Hong Kong, Seoul, Singapore, Tokyo, Taipei, Kuala Lumpur, Sydney, Melbourne and London. It was no accident that the first reported case of infection outside of China was in Thailand. Leung and his team calculated that human-to-human spread of SARS-CoV-2 was already taking place in multiple Chinese cities. Worse, though, they warned that, 'on the present trajectory, [SARS-CoV-2] could be about to become a global epidemic in the absence of mitigation.' They recommended that, 'To possibly succeed [in preventing a pandemic], substantial, even draconian measures that limit population mobility should be seriously and immediately considered in affected areas, as should strategies to drastically reduce within-population contact rates through cancellation of mass gatherings, school closures, and instituting working-from-home arrangements . . .'

They urged the closing of live-animal markets and the acceleration of vaccine development. And they exhorted that 'preparedness plans should be readied for deployment at short notice, including securing supply chains of pharmaceuticals, personal protective equipment, hospital supplies, and the necessary human resources to deal with the consequences of a global outbreak of this magnitude.'[3] Governments had been cautioned.

*

As Adam Kucharski argues in *The Rules of Contagion*, 'If you've seen one pandemic, you've seen . . . one pandemic.'[4] His point is that every pandemic has unique characteristics, which means that generalisations are very hard to make. But there are several crucial features of infections that do reliably influence their propensity to spread.

One critical measure of pandemic potential is the reproduction number, or R_0. This figure represents the expected number of infections produced by a primary case in a completely susceptible population. If the R_0 is 2, then one case becomes two, two becomes four, four becomes eight, and so on. If $R_0 < 1$, the epidemic will eventually die out.

The Wuhan outbreak of SARS-CoV-2 began with an R_0 of around 2.5.[5] That is, it had a high potential for epidemic spread. And spread it did – by direct contact with people who had the infection, including breathing in droplets from the nose or mouth of a person who is infected, or by touching objects or surfaces on which the virus had landed. In a report from the Chinese Center for Disease Control and Prevention describing the early trajectory of the epidemic, Chinese scientists emphasised that 'this novel coronavirus is highly contagious.' They went on,

It has spread extremely rapidly from a single city to the entire country within only about 30 days. Moreover, it has achieved such far-reaching effects even in the face of extreme response measures including the complete shutdown and isolation of whole cities, cancellation of Chinese New Year celebrations, prohibition of attendance at school and work, massive mobilisation of health and public health personnel as well as military medical units, and rapid construction of entire hospitals.[6]

On 23 January, Chinese authorities locked down Wuhan, cutting off all transportation links. Mass quarantine was extended to a total of 36 million people across thirteen additional cities shortly thereafter. But, by then, it was too late. After Thailand, cases transported from Wuhan were reported in Japan, South Korea, the US, Canada, Nepal, Hong Kong, Singapore, Malaysia and Taiwan. The virus tracked rail and air transportation routes out of Wuhan.

The first European cases arrived in France on 24 January, in Germany, on 27 January. The first cases in the UK were described on 31 January. The first death outside China took place in the Philippines on 2 February. On 3 February, the cruise ship *Diamond Princess* was quarantined off Yokohama, Japan. A viral fire had been ignited and it was spreading unchecked around the world.

Italy endured the first humanitarian catastrophe outside of China. The country went into a nationwide lockdown on 9 March. The entire Lombardy region (16 million people) was placed in quarantine. If you left home, you had to carry a certificate explaining the reason for your excursion. Those who violated the lockdown faced fines of between €400 and €3,000.

Spain also suffered an unspeakably traumatic epidemic. The

country went into lockdown on 14 March. France (full) and Germany (partial) implemented lockdowns shortly after – on 17 March and 22 March, respectively. The UK was slower than some of its European neighbours but eventually switched off its economy on 24 March. Days mattered because the epidemic was doubling every forty-eight to seventy-two hours. The British public already knew what was coming. They had begun to change their behaviour well before lockdown became official government policy. UK politicians were behind the public curve, despite being warned by scientists in early March of the threat facing the country. On 27 March, Prime Minister Boris Johnson announced that he too had contracted the infection.

The response in the US was predictably unpredictable. The first imported case was reported from Washington state on 21 January. President Trump initially called SARS-CoV-2 'the new hoax'. By 30 January, he was describing the epidemic as 'pretty much under control'. By 2 February, his administration had 'pretty much shut it down.' By 27 February, 'it will disappear.' On 4 March, he claimed there were 'very small numbers in the US'. 10 March: 'It's really working out.' 12 March: 'It's going to go away.' But, by 17 March, President Trump was forced to admit – 'This is a pandemic.'

Indeed, WHO had declared COVID-19 a pandemic on 11 March. Dr Tedros, by now clearly agitated by the growing global emergency, called 'for countries to take urgent and aggressive action.' 'We cannot say this loudly enough or clearly enough or often enough', he went on; 'all countries can still change the course of this pandemic' if they 'detect, test, treat, isolate, trace, and mobilise their people in the response.' He stressed that 'the challenge for many countries who are now dealing with large clusters or community transmission is not whether they can do the same – it's whether they will.'

Nowhere was spared. WHO reported that 213 countries, areas or territories were affected, from India to Indonesia, from Turkey to Algeria, and from Brazil to Ecuador. No country tested every member of its population, so it is impossible to be precise about the exact number of infections that took place worldwide. Deaths are a more reliable measure, since in many countries there are more formal means of death certification which can be assembled into national mortality statistics. But, even using deaths as a metric, one should be concerned and cautious about the accuracy of data – such as those from Russia, Iran and even China.

China revised its numbers upwards by 50 per cent in April, adding a further 1,290 fatalities to the total reported for Wuhan. And even then it is likely that the total number of deaths reported for China is an underestimate. When account was taken of the changing case definitions China used as its epidemic evolved, one study put the total number of cases at 232,000.

*

At the time of writing (1 January 2021), the number of confirmed cases of SARS-CoV-2 stood at 81,947,503. The total number of reported deaths was 1,808,041. The ten nations with most deaths, as reported by WHO, were:

US	335,789	UK	73,512
Brazil	193,875	France	64,254
India	148,994	Russia	57,555
Mexico	124,897	Iran	55,223
Italy	74,159	Spain	50,442

The global distribution of infection has been highly uneven. As of 1 January 2021, the Americas had recorded 35,511,445 cases of SARS-CoV-2. Europe was not far behind, with 26,490,355 cases. Then came South-East Asia (11,993,294 cases), the Arab world (4,934,617 cases) and Africa (1,919,903 cases). The part of the world where the pandemic began – the Western Pacific region – has so far had the fewest deaths: 1,097,144, a fact not without some tragic irony.

The public health response to this highly contagious virus – the so-called non-pharmaceutical interventions – was initially implemented reluctantly in most Western democracies, and even then in stutteringly incremental steps. First came advice to wash hands regularly and properly (singing 'Happy Birthday' twice), improve cough etiquette, avoid touching your face, and use and then dispose of paper tissues. Next came a recommendation to practise physical distancing and reduce social mixing – at a minimum, avoid shaking hands, hugging, or kissing non-family members. Finally, lockdown – the almost complete closure of entire cultures.

School terms ended abruptly. Universities sent students home. Restaurants put up their shutters. Theatres cancelled productions. Museums locked their doors. Not even local libraries and churches were exempted. Weddings, baptisms and sporting events were all banned. The only retail businesses allowed to remain open were pharmacies, food and hardware stores, supermarkets, petrol stations, bicycle shops, launderettes, garages, car rentals, pet shops, newsagents, post offices and banks. The only reasons you were allowed to leave home, unless you were a key worker (in health and social care, education and childcare, food and necessary goods, local and national government, utilities, public safety and national security, and transport), were to buy essential necessities (as infrequently as possible), visit a doctor or vulnerable person, donate blood, and exercise once a day.

But although the decision to go into full lockdown was hard, it was even harder to decide how to return society to some semblance of normal functioning. In the UK, just three weeks into its lockdown, public debate was already focusing on an exit strategy. But, without either a vaccine to confer immunity or adequate capacity to test, trace and isolate contacts, the prospects for an early exit were nothing more than speculation mixed with touches of fantasy and delusion.

The evidence from Wuhan was sobering.[7] Around 90 per cent of the workforce had been locked down. Assuming an R_0 of over 2 and with a phased return to work (25 per cent of the workforce returning during the two weeks after lockdown ends, then 50 per cent during the next two weeks, and finally 100 per cent returning to work), epidemiologists from the London School of Hygiene and Tropical Medicine calculated that it would be safe to start lifting intense physical distancing measures only in early April. If lockdown was lifted either prematurely or completely, the risk of a second wave of infection flaring up was almost guaranteed.

Since Wuhan's lockdown began on 23 January, that meant at least ten weeks of the most extreme measures to extinguish virus transmission. Wuhan did cautiously start lifting its restrictions on social mixing on 8 April. But many schools, shops and cinemas remained closed.

Gabriel Leung, who correctly predicted that a global pandemic would ensue from the events in Wuhan, was working intensively to define what an exit strategy should look like.[8] He and his team in Hong Kong warned against relaxing restrictions too soon. If the R_0 crept above 1 again, a second wave of the pandemic would be inevitable. He advised resuming economic activity in lockdown settings under what he called an $R<1$ constraint. He also advised continuous surveillance of two critical measures – the Case Fatality Risk and Rt (the instantaneous or effective reproduction number, or the R value at a particular time and place).

The Case Fatality Risk is the ratio of laboratory-confirmed deaths to confirmed cases. It will vary according to the pre-existing levels of health of a population and the availability of healthcare resources. It could be a valuable measure of the health system's ability to treat severe cases of the infection.

Rt would be a sensitive indicator to tell whether the epidemic is resurfacing. Real-time monitoring of Rt will depend on implementing community testing for the early detection of infection, with subsequent contact tracing if someone is found to have the virus, and then quarantine to prevent possible further transmission. Digital monitoring of levels of social mixing could also be helpful.

But maybe the truth is that life will never completely return to normal until vaccines are fully rolled out and herd immunity is achieved – and perhaps not even then. A vaccine is not a 'magic bullet'. It is unlikely to be completely effective, and it is unlikely to be taken up by every citizen. The risk of outbreaks of new clusters from imported cases is likely to be always with us. Perhaps COVID-19 represents an impermeable boundary between one moment in our lives and another. We can never go back.

*

If human life has been so affected, so acutely and so suddenly by this coronavirus, it seems important to ask what the political, economic, social and cultural consequences might be. It is too soon to be sure, of course. But, even while the pandemic was raging through countries, some fiery judgements were being made nevertheless.

David Nabarro, WHO's special envoy for COVID-19, announced with considerable drama on 13 April, 'This virus isn't going to go away . . . Yes, we will have to wear masks. There will be more physical distancing . . . It's a revolution.'

Lockdown has certainly changed the way we interacted with one another. Walking down the street we may cross the road if we see someone else walking towards us. We want to maintain our 1- to 2-metre separation. We queue on the road to get into the supermarket, sometimes waiting over an hour before being allowed to enter. Numbers of shoppers are strictly limited in each store. And we are now used to seeing our fellow citizens wearing masks and rubber gloves. They may back away from us if we come too close or dive into another shopping aisle if we inadvertently turn into their path. Everyone is potentially infected and so everyone is a risk. We can only rely on the safety of our immediate household.

Were these new behaviours simply examples of wise caution at a time of danger? Or did they represent a catastrophic loss of social trust, a fissuring in our communities, a fragmentation of our solidarity? Is that the revolution we have to look forward to?

One revolution certainly did take place – in our working lives. For some of us, the fortunate ones, those who didn't have to earn our living on the frontlines of risk, home – the kitchen table, the sofa or even the bed – became our new office. While working from home might have attractions, the degree of isolation we have lived with has had important implications for mental health.

Samantha Brooks and her colleagues at the Department of Psychological Medicine, King's College London, have reviewed the world literature on the impacts of quarantine. Their findings are alarming.[9] Isolation can cause post-traumatic stress, confusion, fear, anger, frustration and, of course, boredom. Some of these effects will be long-lasting. They have recommended that periods of isolation should be as short as possible. Working from home might be a welcome pleasure at first. But it also carries the seeds of sometimes severe mental trauma.

Democracy also shifted. Parliaments were suspended. Politicians often deployed war-like language ('We are at war with an invisible killer'), with invocations to 'pull together', conjure up our 'Dunkirk sprit' and 'fight' the virus.

War metaphors carry huge emotional force. They are widely understood by the public. Words of war convey a sense of threat, urgency and risk. They suggest a battle with an evil enemy. The stakes are high. Sacrifices will have to be made. But war metaphors have their own dangers. They can create an atmosphere where dissent and criticism of government policy are discouraged, possibly even branded as a kind of betrayal. They emphasise treatment, not prevention. Turning the strategy to tackle a disease into a battlefield could worsen the mental health of those caught in the middle of the 'war zone'. And the idea of war also implies victory or defeat – where neither may be the likely outcome with a virus that is here to stay.

China became a particular focus for comment. Some heaped praise on China's response to SARS-CoV-2. 'We appreciate the seriousness with which China is taking this outbreak,' said Dr Tedros on 28 January. Controversially, he has continued to thank the Chinese government for taking 'action massively at the epicentre, at the source of the outbreak . . . and that helped in preventing cases from being exported to other provinces in China and the rest of the world.'

But others have been less happy with China's tactics. Tom Tugendhat is a British Conservative MP who chairs the influential Parliamentary Foreign Affairs Select Committee. He was scathing about China's coronavirus response. On 13 April, as Wuhan opened up and as the UK was passing through the peak of its deaths, he commented that 'China has deliberately lied in order to preserve the strength of the [Communist] Party at the expense of its people.'

The verdict on the virtues of China's response remains to be written. There are legitimate questions the Chinese government must answer. There is a gap in the timeline of the pandemic outbreak. The earliest known cases reported in China were first described on 1 December 2019. Beijing disclosed the fact of the outbreak on 31 December. What happened during the intervening period? What really took place in Wuhan in December? Did local Communist Party officials suppress evidence of a new virus? Did they delay telling the national government in Beijing? Also, why did Chinese authorities tell WHO on 11–12 January that no additional cases of COVID-19 had been detected since 3 January? That statement was plainly untrue. Was Beijing complicit in playing down the significance of the outbreak? And did China use this time of global turbulence to tighten its grip on territories it has long regarded as within its sphere of influence. On 30 June, the Standing Committee of the National People's Congress enacted the Hong Kong National Security Law, which had a chilling effect on Hong Kong's democracy movement. In December 2020, democracy activists Joshua Wong, Agnes Chow and Ivan Lam all received jail sentences for their involvement in protests in 2019. The Chinese government refutes all criticism.

On 2 February, I received an email entitled 'A desperate plea from an ordinary citizen in China'. The writer called herself Moona. This is what she wrote about living in China during the time of coronavirus:

Currently, there are at least five cities, including Wuhan, that have suspended the public transport system; ten provinces and cities, including Hubei and Beijing, that have shut down road passenger transport; 16 provinces that have suspended inter-provincial passenger transport; and many cities in 28 provinces that have completely or partially suspended urban public transportation. Yesterday, Huanggang issued a notice ordering a house quarantine for all urban households, allowing only a designated family member to shop for essentials once in every two days. The news and constant updates include messages from my local government telling me that many cities have made it mandatory to wear a mask in public or for using public transport. But masks have sold out so quickly in many smaller cities (and online as well), while prices have gone up twenty times. In short, if you are poor, you're more than likely to not get a mask at all – and it's usually the poor who cannot afford to stop working.

At 7:30 pm yesterday, Hangzhou became the first city in China to issue a free mask policy for its citizens in seven urban districts to alleviate the problem that has been the elephant in the room, with an online reservation system for five masks for each person every ten days. Even Wuhan hasn't implemented any government policy like this to help its citizens. So access to masks largely depends on donations and self-help by local communities. The bottom line is, a large population in China is suffering, not just from the virus but from the resulting isolation, high uncertainty, anxiety and stress, reduced resources and freedom for daily living, and loss of income. And the point on income really should be considered. With weak social protection in China, in conjunction with the estimate of 60% of labour engaged in the informal economy in Asian and Pacific developing countries, lack of employment benefits and protection renders people extremely vulnerable to crises, such as the current one. There would have been social outcries if this happened in any other Western country, but just because there isn't an outcry in China doesn't make its people lesser people who shouldn't be treated any less. If anything, it shows how deeply the population has been culturally and politically suppressed, and how the voice of the really poor in China gets completely buried and forgotten. This just isn't right.

In a crisis like this, it hurts me so much to see that it's (once again) the well-off who get priority and consideration. Those who actually do not have the ability or resources to take care of themselves inevitably get left behind. Government policies are understandably a combination of politics, economics, sociology, and international relations. But equality to health gets thrown out of the picture in the middle of all these, even in scholarship. This cannot be right. The top health journals should be redirected toward a more compassionate and sensitive discourse. *The Lancet* please do something, somebody please do something. In a practical sense, the government cares about its 'face' more than anything; if there was a prominent international voice calling for it to look into something it just might . . . and that's all that the suppressed and the poor have for hope. So please, help. I understand this might be an effort in vain, but I really hope it is not. So here it is, a desperate plea, and I really hope this message sees you in good time.

The Chinese government owes the world a more detailed explanation of what took place in Wuhan. I don't mind what we call it – an international inquiry, a fact-finding mission, truth and reconciliation. I don't seek blame. I don't want punishment. I simply want to know what happened. Something happened. We need to know so that we have the best chance of preventing it from happening again. An Independent Panel for Pandemic Preparedness and Response has been convened by WHO to answer these questions. It is chaired by the former prime minister of New Zealand, Helen Clark, and the former president of Liberia, Ellen Johnson Sirleaf. The final report of the panel is to be published in 2021. *The Lancet* also established a COVID-19 Commission in July 2020, led by the economist Jeff Sachs. Its Interim Statement concluded that 'SARS-CoV-2 is a naturally occurring virus rather than the result of laboratory creation and release.'[10] The commission plans to publish two further reports in 2021. Whether the WHO or *The Lancet* initiatives can discover the full truth about the origins of the pandemic and the events of those early weeks remains to be seen.

But whatever the questions about the Chinese government's actions, I also believe we must say this – Chinese scientists and health workers deserve our gratitude. I know from my own knowledge of these dedicated individuals that they worked tirelessly to understand the nature of this pandemic. They made it their duty to work with WHO when they were sure there was reason for global alarm. And, in my dealings with Chinese scientists and policymakers, I have observed nothing less than an extraordinary commitment to collaborate openly and unconditionally to control this disease.

*

Despite the uncertainties – and there are many, since we are still, one year on, in the early phase of understanding this disease – perhaps we do know enough to draw two conclusions.

First, much attention was given to the celebrities who contracted SARS-CoV-2 – Marianne Faithfull, Tom Hanks and Rita Wilson, Idris Elba, Sophie Trudeau, Prince Albert of Monaco, Prince Charles in the UK, Plácido Domingo, Jackson Browne, George Stephanopoulos, Bryan Cranston, Antonio Banderas, Brian Cox, Kanye West. It was easy to think the virus was a threat to everyone equally. But that was not the case. COVID-19 overwhelmingly affected those who were poorer, less able and sicker. There was a steep social gradient to this disease. And it seemed to affect black and minority ethnic communities especially badly. Those on the frontlines of care were particularly vulnerable and often unprotected. COVID-19 exploited and worsened already existing inequalities in society. Second, before COVID-19, the idea of a 'key worker' was probably a rather obscure notion in the public's mind. No longer. Just as 'first responders' after 9/11 – firefighters, police officers and emergency medical workers – became heroic symbols of a country under terrorist attack, so key workers came to embody the commitment of those without whom society really would have collapsed.

The essential services key workers provide – whether they were health workers dispensing care, people working in supermarkets ensuring continuous supplies of food, or those delivering vital services, from refuse collection to public utilities – became the resilient and moral backbone of the response worldwide. It was these key workers who kept countries going while the rest of us languished at home. It was these key workers who saved the lives of the sick and protected the lives of the poor and vulnerable. It was these key workers, so often overlooked and taken for granted, who, as we now realised, were and are the real foundation for public order and public safety in our societies. We truly do owe them our lives.

Why Were We Not Prepared?

We need to accept that the timing of a disaster's occurrence is unambiguously random.

Lucy Jones, *The Big Ones* (2018)

'We were poorly prepared.' Ian Boyd was writing in *Nature* in March 2020.[1] He had been one of the UK government's chief scientific advisers from 2012 to 2019 and recalled taking part in a 'practice run' for an influenza pandemic. 200,000 people died in this simulation. 'It left me shattered.' Did government learn from this experiment to identify critical weaknesses in the national response to an epidemic? Boyd notes, ruefully, 'We learnt what would help, but did not necessarily implement those lessons.'

Boyd was alluding to Exercise Cygnus – scenario planning for a pandemic influenza outbreak that took place in October 2016. Pandemic influenza is top of the UK government's National Risk Register. A pandemic is deemed the most severe civil emergency risk to our society. The same is true for most Western democracies. The result of Cygnus was a stark warning: UK preparedness was 'currently not sufficient to cope with the extreme demands of a severe epidemic.'

National failings were sometimes sublimated into international attacks. In a remarkable speech given at the White House on 14 April, President Donald Trump issued an instruction 'to halt funding of the World Health Organization while a review is conducted to assess the World Health Organization's role in severely mismanaging and covering up the spread of the coronavirus.' This was an astonishing allegation. An American president was charging WHO with nothing less than murder – 'so much death has been caused by their mistakes.' His case against WHO was incendiary and is worth quoting at length. The speech will become a key document in the history of antagonism, recrimination and blame that marked so much of this pandemic.

One of the most dangerous and costly decisions from the WHO was its disastrous decision to oppose travel restrictions from China and other nations . . . The WHO's attack on travel restrictions put political correctness above life-saving measures . . . The reality is that the WHO failed to adequately obtain, vet, and share information in a timely and transparent fashion . . . The WHO failed in this basic duty and must be held accountable . . . The WHO failed to investigate credible reports from sources in Wuhan that conflicted directly with the Chinese government's official accounts. There was credible information to suspect human-to-human transmission in December, 2019, which should have spurred the WHO to investigate and investigate immediately. Through the middle of January it parroted and publicly endorsed the idea that there was not human-to-human transmission happening, despite reports and clear evidence to the contrary. The delays that WHO experienced in declaring a public health emergency cost valuable time ... The inability of the WHO to obtain virus samples to this date has deprived the scientific community of essential data ... Had the WHO done its job to get medical experts into China to objectively assess the situation on the ground and to call out China's lack of transparency the outbreak could have been contained at its source with very little death, very little death, and certainly very little death by comparison. This would have saved thousands of lives and avoided worldwide economic damage. Instead, the WHO willingly took China's assurances at face value and ... defended the actions of the Chinese government, even praising China for its so-called transparency – I don't think so. The WHO pushed China's misinformation about the virus, saying it was not communicable and there was no need for travel bans ... The WHO's reliance on China's disclosures likely caused a twenty-fold increase in cases worldwide and it may be much more than that. The WHO has not addressed a single one of these concerns nor provided a serious explanation that acknowledges its own mistakes of which there were many.

So many statements in this speech are factually incorrect. There was no credible information available to WHO in December 2019 about the Wuhan outbreak, and certainly no evidence about person-to-person transmission. WHO did not fail to obtain, vet or share information in a timely or transparent fashion. On the contrary, it acted immediately to investigate the first published notice about the outbreak. Once the agency's officials had verified that there was indeed an outbreak of a novel pneumonia, they acted quickly to alert other countries. In January, WHO did not deny that the virus could be transmitted from person to person. The organisation was careful to confirm that this means of transmission was possible before saying so publicly – an appropriately scientific position to take. Finally, WHO did not push 'China's misinformation about the virus'. It established its own robust investigatory procedures to gather information so that it could declare a Public Health Emergency of International Concern on 30 January. In my thirty years as an editor at *The Lancet* I have never seen a political leader lie so comprehensively to the public.

I believe that President Trump's decision to cut funding to WHO in the middle of a global pandemic was so egregious that it constituted a crime against humanity. Is that claim an exaggeration? I don't believe so, and here is why. WHO exists to protect the health and wellbeing of the world's peoples. A crime against humanity is a knowing and inhumane attack against a people. By attacking and weakening WHO while the agency was doing all it could to protect individuals in some of the most vulnerable countries in the world, President Trump has, in my view, met the criteria for an act of violence the international community calls a crime against humanity.

*

So who was responsible for a pandemic that infected over 80 million people and killed over 1.8 million? China? National governments? WHO? Some of the answers, I think, lie in the lessons from the last outbreak of a SARS virus in 2002–3.

In late 2002 in the southern Chinese province of Guangdong, a new coronavirus jumped from its animal host into humans. That event most likely took place in a live-animal market where a multiplicity of animals were caged, slaughtered, dismembered, and sold raw and cooked. These markets are crowded, busy and atrociously unhygienic. The likelihood of a virus making the transition from animal to human is high. The first known person to acquire the virus and to develop the associated disease it caused in November 2002 – an unusual type of pneumonia, the 'index case' – was from the city of Foshan.

Further outbreaks were reported in December. A Chinese team of scientists concluded in January 2003 that a new virus was probably responsible. They urged careful surveillance and reporting. But because their recommendations coincided with Chinese New Year they were either ignored or neglected. Not only was China's guard down, but the enormous numbers of people travelling home for New Year celebrations provided the perfect opportunity for the virus to spread. Which it did.

On 31 January in Guangzhou, a patient, ill and infected with this new virus, was admitted to one and then transferred to two further hospitals, passing the infection to around 200 people. As the number of those infected grew, news reached WHO. The agency's officials asked the Chinese government for details. They were told there was an outbreak of an acute respiratory illness that had affected 305 people, with five deaths.

Hong Kong suffered an outbreak of the new disease too. Twelve people staying at the Metropole Hotel fell sick with SARS in February 2003. They had contracted the virus from an infected doctor visiting from the Chinese mainland. Those twelve individuals returned home with the virus – to Singapore, Vietnam, Canada, Ireland and the US. Most of the more than 8,000 cases worldwide originated from this superspreading moment. In March 2003, more than 300 people fell ill in the Amoy Gardens apartment towers.

By 12 March, under the leadership of the former Norwegian prime minister Gro Harlem Brundtland, WHO had issued a global alert. The responses from the affected countries were fast and impressive. Strict containment led to the extinguishing of the outbreak by May 2003. This particular coronavirus hasn't re-emerged since.

The outbreak was short, sharp and, although global, strictly confined to a very limited number of countries. But its effects had huge consequences. First, there was an enormous economic shock. Estimates put the short-term cost at US$80 billion, with China and Hong Kong especially badly hit. Second, there were implications for global health security. Health was no longer a minor or marginal political issue. Strengthening health systems now became a matter of national defence and homeland security.

A further lesson was that epidemics such as SARS had to be fought internationally, as well as locally. The response to a virus that can spread so fast and furiously cannot be haphazard. It has to be coordinated. But the most cataclysmic lesson was political.

China performed poorly. The country's weak public health and primary healthcare systems, its turgid and authoritarian bureaucracy, excessive respect for political hierarchy, poor coordination, suppression of evidence, repression of the media, reluctance to ask for external assistance, and fear of internal instability all contributed to a less than optimal response. Chinese officials simply refused to share information with WHO. They practised a systematic deception.

On 16 April, WHO expressed 'strong concern over inadequate reporting' of SARS cases. It is extremely rare for WHO to criticise one of its member states. But Brundtland's frustration was growing and, as a former prime minister, she had the confidence to call out the Chinese government. By 20 April 2003, China's minister of health and Beijing's mayor had both been fired by the new Chinese president, Hu Jintao. The government declared a 'nationwide war on SARS'. They vowed never to be shamed in the same way again.

The global response to SARS was judged a glorious success. By July, WHO was able to declare that the virus had been vanquished. As the respected US Institute of Medicine (IOM) concluded in 2004, 'the quality, speed, and effectiveness of the public health response to SARS brilliantly outshone past responses to international outbreaks of infectious disease, validating a decade's worth of progress in global public health networking.'[2]

This sense of achievement was matched with a warning. The IOM noted that SARS 'highlights the continuing need for investments in a robust response system that is prepared for the next emerging disease – whether naturally occurring or intentionally introduced.' Brundtland concluded that 'This is not the time to relax our vigilance. The world must remain on high alert for cases of SARS.'

The risk of a virally induced global humanitarian emergency was identified as a clear and present danger after SARS. The future required countries to build defences against a re-emergence of the virus – indeed, to prepare the world for the next pandemic of whatever kind. The most important demand was vigilance – a heightened and permanent state of awareness. Practically, there must be a scientific readiness to identify the agent causing an outbreak, develop diagnostic tests, and discover new medicines and vaccines that could treat and eventually prevent the disease. The public health response that was needed was also clear – surveillance, early detection, isolation, contact tracing, quarantine, accumulating surge capacity within the health system to cope with what might be tens of thousands of severe infections, and effective communication to the public. Modern quarantine means reducing the frequency of social contact, voluntary home curfew, cancelling mass gatherings, avoiding public transport, and closing public buildings and workplaces. These measures would introduce severe and unusual restrictions on the lives of most citizens. To win public acceptance, it would be essential to establish trust through rapid, regular and transparent communication, protect living standards through the provision of job security and compensation schemes, and maintain the morale of key workers. Finally, it was necessary to understand that SARS was 'a watershed event in the history of public health because of the degree of multinational cooperation to contain the disease'.[3]

Indeed, SARS represented the beginning of an entirely new geopolitical era. As noted by David Fidler, a specialist in international relations and global health law, 'SARS represents the first infectious disease to emerge into a radically new and different global political environment for public health.'[4] The 'historic moment' that was SARS came about because the coronavirus was 'the first post-Westphalian pathogen'.

The Peace of Westphalia in 1648 not only ended the Thirty Years' War but also initiated the birth of the modern nation-state. From 1648 until 2002–3, infectious diseases – indeed, all disease – were managed largely within the confines of national borders. For over three centuries international relations were shaped by three principles: national sovereignty, non-intervention in the affairs of sovereign states, and consent-based international law.

Fidler described Westphalian governance as horizontal. It involved only states, focusing mainly on the details of how states should interact with one another. It made no attempt to address the way governments treated their own peoples. Countries might work together to strengthen their own national plans for tackling disease – for example, through the technical committees and resolutions passed at annual World Health Assemblies – but SARS was the first occasion when sovereign states had to bend to the influence of non-state actors and global organisations, such as WHO.

Just as science, from Copernicus through Darwin to Einstein, has been an exercise in the gradual erosion of human vanity – the decentring of the human being from our understanding of the world – so pandemics have eroded governmental omnipotence. Nation-states have slowly had to succumb to curbs on their power and authority.

SARS was a different kind of pathogen because, like HIV, it posed a truly global threat. It became a global public health emergency. SARS inaugurated a new era of post-Westphalian public health – public health that transcended national borders and national sovereignties. And that new era itself was inaugurated with an achievement of spectacular proportions: 'the global campaign against SARS achieved a victory that will go down in the annals of public health and international relations history.'

Since SARS, there have been two further major outbreaks of zoonotic disease. One was Ebola in 2013. Countries and global agencies displayed disgraceful complacency in their lacklustre response to Ebola. A year earlier, another coronavirus – causing the Middle-East Respiratory Syndrome – hit Saudi Arabia and spread to Qatar and several other countries in the Arab world. Thankfully, the risk of person-to-person transmission was low and so MERS did not become the global threat that both SARS and Ebola posed. The world was not tested by MERS.

Zika was a different story. Transmitted by the bite of an infected *Aedes* mosquito and beginning in early 2015, Zika virus is suspected to have infected over half a million people, with most cases being reported in Brazil, Colombia, Venezuela, Martinique and Honduras. In February 2016, WHO declared a PHEIC in response to Zika virus. The epidemic ended in November 2016. But the tragedy of Zika is that the virus can be passed from a pregnant woman to her foetus, thereby causing an array of birth defects, notably microcephaly.

By the end of the West African Ebola and the Zika outbreaks in 2016, there was ample evidence to signal the urgent need for countries to strengthen their preparedness for new infectious pandemics. But, as WHO has described, fewer than half the countries of the world have the public health capacity to prevent or respond to new outbreaks of disease.[5] Any weak link in the global chain of preparedness and protection is a threat to all countries.

WHO warned, 'Many countries are struggling to sustain or develop their national preparedness capacities, primarily because of a lack of resources, competing national priorities, and a high turnover of health-care workers . . . Urgent action is needed to ensure that capacities are in place to prevent and manage health emergencies.' But these weaknesses were not addressed or prioritised by most nations. Even countries that were relatively well resourced – countries such as Italy, for example – found themselves engulfed by the consequences of SARS-CoV-2. Partly, this failure to react to the threat can be explained by an understandable fear of the economic consequences of lockdowns. 'Milan does not stop,' said the mayor of Milan, Beppe Sala.

But the most important reason for the widespread complacency across much of Europe and North America was that political leaders underestimated the danger. They could not believe that a virus that originated in a Chinese city they had probably never heard of could have such calamitous effects in their own communities. Despite all of the evidence pointing to the devastating damage of recent infectious epidemics, this risk was just not on their horizon of possibilities.

The fact that this was so points to a miserable failure of government. Some political leaders have accepted and admitted these failures. As President Macron said on 13 April 2020, 'Were we ready? Obviously, not enough.'

In many countries, this lack of political vigilance was compounded by a decade of austerity economics that followed the global financial crisis of 2007–8. The Great Recession that ensued was one of the most severe downturns in the global economy since the Great Depression of the 1930s. Policies of austerity led to squeezed government budgets. And the health sector was often a particular victim of cuts in social spending.

In the UK after 2010, the National Health Service (NHS) saw an unprecedented decline in its growth at the same time as patient demand was increasing. Britain's public health system has endured £1 billion of cuts since 2015. Worse, the local infrastructure of public health, so essential for protecting communities from infection, was dismantled.

This reduction in growth in health spending was felt across most of Europe. Health services became steadily understaffed, short of resources, and stretched to breaking point, especially during winter months when patient demand was at its highest. In the decade leading up to COVID-19, the capacity of health systems could not keep pace with growing populations, ageing societies, changing patterns of disease and more expensive new treatments.

Despite President Trump's attempt to blame WHO and China for the destructive effects of COVID-19 on American society, it was the lack of readiness of the US public healthcare system that played a more important part. Public health departments nationally, in states and locally have been chronically underfunded. The Trump administration specifically targeted the US Centers for Disease Control and Prevention. Its budget was savaged, reducing epidemic prevention efforts across the world, including in China. The position of White House director for global health security and biothreats was axed by John Bolton, then national security advisor, in 2019, leaving no one to identify and call out the dangers of a global pandemic. The US was spectacularly unprepared for SARS-CoV-2, largely owing to its own acts of self-harm.

These turns away from investment in national and global health security reflect a larger trend: a general political antipathy to globalism – that is, an appreciation of the importance of international interdependence, solidarity and cooperation between nations and peoples. A decade of austerity created the conditions for politicians and their electorates to look inwards. Attending to the predicaments of one's own country is no bad thing. But there was a larger ideology at work.

Donald Trump in America, Brexit in the UK, Jair Bolsonaro in Brazil, Narendra Modi in India, Italy's Five Star Movement – each of these political watersheds stood for a departure from what had been, until the global financial crisis, a steady political alignment around a common global story: the need for greater international collaboration to solve some of the world's most pressing problems.

In the words of President Trump, speaking at the United Nations General Assembly in 2018, 'We reject the ideology of globalism, and we embrace the doctrine of patriotism.' And again, in 2019, 'The future does not belong to globalists, the future belongs to patriots.' But this narrow definition of patriotism ignored one brutal truth: viruses have no nationality.

The result of this turn away from globalism is that when SARS-CoV-2 arrived there was no global leadership, no willingness to cooperate, and no ability to view what was taking place as a lethal global challenge demanding a coordinated global response. Instead, there was inattention, rivalry and accusation.

*

This brittle and dysfunctional 'international community' was also unprepared for a second epidemic – what has come to be called by WHO an 'infodemic'. An infodemic is an overflow of information, some of it true, some of it not, which hampers a reliable and effective response to an epidemic. When confronted by a plethora of claims and counter-claims, who should one believe?

There have been debilitating examples of misinformation throughout the SARS-CoV-2 outbreak. These fall into four categories – first, conflicting theories about the cause of the disease. The view that this virus emerged as a zoonotic infection from a live-animal market in Wuhan has been challenged by several theories. The most conspiratorial is the claim that the virus was somehow engineered and then leaked from a biological weapons facility in the city. President Trump gave credence to the idea in April when he said, 'More and more we're hearing the story . . . We'll see.' Distracting attention away from the dangers of live-animal markets will only diminish the pressure to close those markets down. Another theory was that 5G wireless technology damaged human immune systems, thereby contributing to severe COVID-19 illness. 5G masts have been attacked and burnt down as a result. WHO has ruled that 5G signals pose no risk to human health, but still the idea persists.

A second source of misinformation concerns the symptoms of the illness and how the virus is transmitted. In India, some Hindu nationalists have sought to argue, incorrectly, that the Muslim community had tried to spread the virus deliberately to the Hindu population. They coined the terms 'corona-terrorism' and 'corona-Jihad', inciting discrimination, harassment and violence against Indian Muslims. Chinese citizens have also experienced overt racism and xenophobia, not helped by President Trump calling SARS-CoV-2 the 'Wuhan virus' and 'the plague from China'.

The third category of misinformation relates to alleged COVID-19 cures. There are by now hundreds of false stories of tests and treatments for this disease, including vitamin C, cocaine, marijuana and colloidal silver. And, finally, questions have been raised about what health authorities are doing to tackle the pandemic. One theory, widely circulated, has been that COVID-19 is largely an invention by the media and that the disease is no worse than a routine influenza epidemic – emphatically untrue.

WHO became so worried about the effects of an infodemic that it established a new unit – the Information Network for Epidemics, or EPI-WIN – to counter its impact.

But what is more sinister still is the part disinformation might have played in propagating false beliefs about COVID-19. Disinformation is that category of misinformation deliberately aimed to deceive. Those who propagate disinformation seek to amplify discord within societies. The European External Action Service has documented multiple examples of disinformation targeted at Europe and the European Union (EU). The intention behind these attacks is often to discredit the EU for the way it has handled the crisis, to suggest that the EU has failed to help its member states, and to show that other countries, such as China, have done more to help Europe than Europe itself. The false theories being distributed are typical, so the European External Action Service argues, of pro-Kremlin propaganda that aims 'to amplify divisions, sow distrust and chaos, and exacerbate crisis situations and issues of public concern.'

The answer as to why the world was unprepared for SARS-CoV-2 and COVID-19 has several further and even more disturbing twists, which I will discuss in the next three chapters. Collectively, these deficiencies in decision-making reflect not only the surprising fragility of modern science-based societies but also something far worse – inherent failures in the mechanics of Western democracies that threaten their very existence.

3

Science: The Paradox of Success and Failure

A catalogue of the number of deaths induced by the major epidemics of historical times is staggering, and dwarfs the total deaths on all past battlefields.

Roy M. Anderson and Robert M. May,
Infectious Diseases of Humans (1991)

The global scientific community made an unrivalled contribution to establishing a reliable foundation of knowledge to guide the response to the SARS-CoV-2 pandemic. And yet the management of COVID-19 represented, in many countries, the greatest science policy failure for a generation. What went wrong?

Before answering this question, one should acknowledge and applaud the successes. After enduring the global opprobrium following its handling of SARS twenty years ago, Chinese leaders invested heavily in their universities, and specifically in their capacities for scientific, technical and medical research. Confronted by a new virus, Chinese scientists were ready, equipped and swung quickly into action.

They reported the first forty-one cases of COVID-19 in *The Lancet* on 24 January. The Chinese team was led by Bin Cao, a professor in the Department of Pulmonary and Critical Care Medicine at the China–Japan Friendship Hospital in Beijing. He assembled groups in Wuhan and Beijing which began to put together the epidemiological, clinical, laboratory and radiological data from this initial group of patients.[1]

Bin Cao and his colleagues provided the first case descriptions of symptoms and signs for COVID-19, an essential and urgent resource for doctors around the world facing patients with an unfamiliar type of pneumonia. They made the connection between the illness and exposure to the live-animal market. They described how a third of patients had to be admitted to intensive care. They calculated the average time from the onset of symptoms to ICU admission (10.5 days). They showed that patients often had blood profiles that revealed serious cardiac, renal and liver injuries. Chest computed tomography produced images that were abnormal in every case, giving the appearance of ground glass throughout the lung fields. One pattern of investigation was particularly disturbing – elevated levels of cytokines that constituted a 'cytokine storm'. The Chinese team described how some patients needed invasive mechanical ventilation and a special means to oxygenate blood when the lungs failed – a technique called extracorporeal membrane oxygenation. They also described how 15 per cent of the patients admitted to hospital had died.

The contrast between this impressive response and China's pitiful efforts during SARS in 2002–3 illustrates the remarkable scientific renaissance that had taken place in the country in just two decades. Bin Cao's team was not only able to gather state-of-the-art data on these early patients but was also encouraged to write up their work, publish it free from censorship in foreign English-language medical journals, and make their findings available to others – all within weeks of the first reports of the new disease. The cultural, as well as the scientific, shift that had taken place in China was monumental. Not that this effort was without controversy at home. Some of the Chinese scientists who wrote the early reports for *The Lancet* were targeted for criticism on Chinese social media. Why, they were asked, did Chinese scientists publish their work in English-language journals and not their Chinese equivalents? Was this not an act of national betrayal? What these allegations of disloyalty failed to understand was that, since the first SARS outbreak in 2002–3, Chinese science has become embedded and integrated into what is a truly international scientific enterprise. Many leading Chinese scientists today have been trained in Western universities. And the Chinese government has lured many of the country's best scientists back to China with offers of well-equipped laboratories, promotion, research funding and high salaries.

Several further milestones were achieved by local scientific teams. Hong Kong clinicians working with colleagues in Shenzhen were the first to establish person-to-person transmission of SARS-CoV-2.[2] The genome sequence of the new virus was published on 29 January by a large team that included China's Center for Disease Control and Prevention, led by its president George Gao (he was one of those accused of treachery by some of his more nationalist compatriots).[3] As I have already discussed, Gabriel Leung's group at the WHO Collaborating Centre for Infectious Disease Epidemiology and Control at the University of Hong Kong carefully documented the likelihood of a global epidemic.[4]

There were several urgent clinical questions that needed to be answered. Again, Chinese clinicians and scientists moved fast. Given the history of Zika virus and its effects on the foetus, one immediate question was whether this coronavirus could be transmitted from mother to baby. Joint teams from Wuhan and Beijing collaborated to study nine pregnant women who had COVID-19. Evidence of intrauterine vertical transmission was assessed by looking for SARS-CoV-2 in amniotic fluid, umbilical cord blood, breast milk and throat swabs from the newly born babies.[5] All women underwent Caesarean section and all survived. And all nine children were born alive and well. None became infected with the virus. None of the samples taken for testing proved positive. Huijun Chen and his colleagues tentatively drew a preliminary but reassuring conclusion – there was no evidence that the virus could pass from mother to baby.

A further concern was the seriousness of COVID-19. The report of the first forty-one patients indicated that one-third required admission to ICU and one in eight died. A report of ninety-nine patients, published on 29 January, described an 11 per cent mortality rate among those admitted to hospital.[6] But more detailed descriptions of the severity of the illness were needed. How much should other countries be worried by this disease?

The early reports indicated that national health systems should be scaling up intensive-care facilities, building stocks of personal protective equipment, and preparing for potentially high mortality. Wuhan's Jin Yin-tan Hospital had been designated a specialist centre to treat patients with COVID-19. A team of doctors led by Professor You Shang reviewed their records and found that, out of 201 patients with confirmed COVID-19, 55 (27 per cent) became so critically ill that they required admission to ICU.[7] As they wrote on 21 February, 'During the outbreak of SARS-CoV-2 infection, the number of critically ill patients exceeded the capacity of ICUs. Therefore, two provisional ICUs were urgently established in Jin Yin-tan hospital.' But what they recorded was shocking – 62 per cent of the patients admitted to ICU died. Those who died were older (their average age was sixty-five) and they developed multiple-organ failure. You Shang concluded that 'The mortality of critically ill patients with SARS-CoV-2 is considerable ... The severity of SARS-CoV-2 pneumonia poses great strain on critical care resources in hospitals, especially if they are not adequately staffed or resourced.' This information was available to Western scientists and clinicians in February, a full month before their countries were forced into lockdown. Again, it remains inexplicable why these reports did not trigger a more urgent and vigorous response from Western governments.

Between 16 and 24 February, a team from WHO visited China to assess the Chinese response to this coronavirus and to offer recommendations for countries not yet affected.[8] They concluded:

In the face of a previously unknown virus, China has rolled out perhaps the most ambitious, agile and aggressive disease containment effort in history . . . Achieving China's exceptional coverage with and adherence to these containment measures has only been possible due to the deep commitment of the Chinese people to collective action in the face of this common threat . . . China's bold approach to contain the rapid spread of this new respiratory pathogen has changed the course of a rapidly escalating and deadly epidemic.

Central to this success was the 'series of major emergency research programs on virus genomics, antivirals, traditional Chinese medicines, clinical trials, vaccines, diagnostics and animal models'. China's commitment to rapidly acquiring knowledge about this new virus was a critical factor in enabling the country to contain, suppress and eventually extinguish the epidemic.

Meanwhile, owing to Wuhan's position as a central Chinese transportation hub, the virus was moving globally. Clinicians reported cases in real time as they arrived in Nepal,[9] Canada,[10] Italy,[11] the US[12] and Singapore.[13] The case of Italy was an especially important example of how science could contribute to a more effective national and international response.

During February, it was becoming clear that Italy was facing an outbreak of unusual force. Giuseppe Remuzzi directs the Mario Negri Institute of Pharmacology Research in Bergamo. As he saw his hospital fill with patients requiring intensive care and ventilation, he began to foresee a humanitarian crisis unfolding. By early March, Italy, and especially the Lombardy region in the north, had seen over 12,000 cases of infection, with 827 deaths. The average age of those who had died was eighty-one, and more than two-thirds of patients had medical histories of diabetes, cancer or heart disease. Remuzzi calculated that Italian hospitals simply did not have the capacity to treat the mass of patients that would present once the first wave of SARS- CoV-2 swept through the country. It was forecast that more than 30,000 Italians would be infected by 15 March.[14] Remuzzi was direct in his conclusions: Italy faced a predicament of 'unmanageable dimensions', one that would have 'catastrophic results'. He predicted that the events that had overwhelmed Hubei would soon engulf Lombardy. The numbers unfortunately supported Remuzzi's worst fears. Italy is in the top five countries to have suffered the highest burden of death from COVID-19.

The story of COVID-19 in the US is one of the strangest paradoxes of the whole pandemic. No other country in the world has the concentration of scientific skill, technical knowledge and productive capacity possessed by the US. It is the world's scientific superpower bar none. And yet this colossus of science utterly failed to bring its expertise successfully to bear on the policy and politics of the nation's response. More people died in the US from COVID-19 in the first three months of the pandemic than during the entire Vietnam War (there were 58,318 US soldiers killed in action in Vietnam between 1955 and 1975; deaths from COVID-19 exceeded that figure on 28 April 2020).

The first case of COVID-19 in the US was reported on 21 January in a young man from Washington state who had returned from Wuhan a week earlier, on 15 January. Nancy Messonnier, who directed America's National Center for Immunization and Respiratory Diseases, called the news 'concerning'.

Commenting on the events unfolding in China, on 24 January President Trump wrote on Twitter that 'It will all turn out well.' Anthony Fauci, the long-standing and much respected director of the National Institute of Allergy and Infectious Diseases, noted, 'We don't want the American public to be worried about this because their risk is low.' But, by 30 January, the US Centers for Disease Control and Prevention reported the country's first case of person-to-person transmission, in a woman whose husband had been in Wuhan. Still, the government assessed the risk to the American public as 'low'.

But by 31 January, the day after WHO declared a PHEIC, President Trump had called coronavirus a public health emergency. Travel bans were implemented. Yet the government still didn't seem to comprehend the urgency and deadliness of the threat. By 12 February, the first American had died of COVID-19. On 21 February, Messonnier agreed that it was now 'very possible' that spread in the community could take place. By the end of February, that possibility became a reality, and Vice-President Mike Pence was appointed by Trump to lead the nation's response to COVID-19.

Pence and Fauci agreed that testing and isolation of those who tested positive should be the cornerstone of their national strategy. But it became clear during March that America's healthcare system, in Fauci's words, was 'not set up for that'. 'That is a failing,' he said. The result was that by the end of March efforts to contain the virus had floundered.

The US had become the most infected nation on the planet. Social distancing and avoiding mass gatherings now became the approved policy of the Trump administration. But the virus had taken hold and deaths began to escalate – as did unemployment as the economy crashed. By May, the US Treasury had announced it was borrowing a record $3 trillion to pay for the coronavirus relief measures passed by Congress.

Wuhan began its lockdown early – on 23 January. Through strenuous efforts to cut the lines of viral transmission, China was able to begin to lift its restrictions on 8 April. As it did so, Deborah Birx, appointed by Pence as the coordinator of the White House coronavirus task force, reported that the epidemic had now reached its peak in the US. By 11 April, the country had surpassed Italy in its number of COVID-19 deaths. Every state had been affected. As the economy imploded further, and as protests broke out about the stay-at-home orders, President Trump turned his fire on China and WHO. On 14 April, he announced that he would stop funding the agency, and he accused China of withholding crucial information about the virus.

The situation in the UK was no less disastrous. From the last week in January, it took the UK government seven weeks to recognise the seriousness of COVID-19. It wasted the whole of February and most of March, when ministers should have been preparing the country for the arrival of a lethal new virus. Why? Inexplicably, medical and scientific advisers to the UK government ignored the warnings coming from China.

Boris Johnson won a general election on 13 December 2019 on the promise that he would 'get Brexit done'. Britain was leaving the European Union on 31 January, a day, the new prime minister said, that symbolised a moment for 'national renewal and change'. On 26 February, less than a month after WHO had declared a PHEIC, he announced an integrated review of foreign policy, defence, security and international development. Johnson claimed this review would be the largest since the Cold War. He spoke about 'the changing nature of threats we face'. But he failed to mention the new coronavirus seeding itself across the country. Did Brexit influence the UK's go-it-alone approach?

By 2 March, Prime Minister Johnson was chairing COBRA, the civil contingencies committee that is convened to handle issues of national emergency. After that meeting, he agreed that COVID-19 presented 'a significant challenge'. 'But we are well-prepared,' he said. Was Johnson aware of Exercise Cygnus, with its clear conclusion in 2016 that the UK was most definitely not well prepared? If he was, he lied to the public. If he was not, then he is surely guilty of misconduct in public office. Remember: a pandemic is top of the UK's National Risk Register. A prime minister should reasonably be expected to understand the capability of his country to address the most severe civil emergency risk.

The best that Prime Minster Johnson could do was advise

hand-washing. He was still arguing that the UK 'remains extremely well-prepared' on 3 March.

On 5 March, when there were eighty-five confirmed cases of COVID-19 in the UK, Johnson went on national television to continue to minimise the risks of the virus. On ITV's *This Morning* he said, 'Perhaps you could sort of take it on the chin, take it all in one go and allow the disease, as it were, to move through the population without really taking as many draconian measures. I think we need to strike a balance.' He displayed his own disregard for the risks of infection by regularly shaking hands with those he met – and bragging about it afterwards.

But by 7 March the government was advising people with symptoms to self-isolate. Ministers seemed unsure of what to do. Let the epidemic rip through the population – 'take it on the chin' – or do something more? By 12 March, the UK had stopped its policy of test, contact trace and isolate – a decision later acknowledged as a mistake. For still unknown reasons, the UK government waited. And watched.

The scientists advising ministers seemed to believe that this new virus could be treated much like influenza. Graham Medley, one of the government's expert scientific advisors, was disarmingly explicit. In an interview on the BBC's television programme *Newsnight*, he explained the UK's early attitude – to encourage a controlled epidemic of large numbers of people in order to generate 'herd immunity'. He recommended 'a situation where the majority of the population are immune to the infection. And the only way of developing that, in the absence of a vaccine, is for the majority of the population to become infected.' Medley advocated 'a nice big epidemic'. 'What we are going to have to try and do', he said, was to 'manage this acquisition of herd immunity and minimise the exposure of people who are vulnerable.' Sir Patrick Vallance, the government's chief scientific advisor, suggested that the goal was to infect 60 per cent of the UK's population.

As March proceeded, government ministers became increasingly anxious. But they were still unable to act decisively. Their staccato decision-making suggested an atmosphere of mounting confusion and fear. On 16 March, the public was advised to cease non-essential travel. On 18 March, schools were closed. And on 20 March, entertainment venues, bars and restaurants were shut. It took until 23 March for the 'stay at home' order to be issued. Critical time had been lost while the epidemic was doubling every two to three days – a fact know to ministers since early March.

What is so mysterious is that it didn't need the predictions of scientists at Imperial College London in March to estimate the impact of a 'watch-and-wait' approach. Any numerate school student could make the calculation. With a mortality of 1 per cent among 60 per cent of a UK population of some 66 million people, the UK could expect almost 400,000 deaths if it took no action. The huge wave of critically ill patients that would result from this strategy of 'take it on the chin' herd immunity would quickly overwhelm the NHS, just as had been the case in Italy. The UK's best scientists had known since the first report from China in January that COVID-19 was a lethal illness. Yet they too did too little, too late.

Remuzzi had also warned European countries. Describing the lessons of his experience in Lombardy, he wrote that 'These considerations might also apply to other European countries that could have similar numbers of patients infected and similar needs regarding intensive care admissions.' And yet the UK continued with its strategy of encouraging the epidemic to tear through communities unchecked.

Nobody can claim ignorance. Nobody can say this interpretation of events is hindsight. Writing in 1994 in her treatise *The Coming Plague*, Laurie Garrett concluded,

> Ultimately, humanity will have to change its perspective on its place in Earth's ecology if the species hopes to stave off or survive the next plague. Rapid globalization of human niches requires that human beings everywhere on the planet go beyond viewing their neighborhoods, provinces, countries, or hemispheres as the sum total of their personal ecospheres. Microbes, and their vectors, recognize none of the artificial boundaries erected by human beings . . . In the microbial world warfare is a constant . . . Time is short.[15]

If you think Garrett's language rhetorical hyperbole, consult the more sober analysis from the US Institute of Medicine in 2004. They evaluated the lessons of the 2003 SARS outbreak, quoting Goethe: 'Knowing is not enough; we must apply. Willing is not enough; we must do.' The Institute of Medicine concluded, 'The rapid containment of SARS is a success in public health, but also a warning . . . If SARS reoccurs . . . health systems worldwide will be put under extreme pressure

. . . Continued vigilance is vital.'[16] But the world ignored these warnings.

Consider these outbreaks: Hendra in 1994, Nipah in 1998, SARS in 2003, MERS in 2012 and Ebola in 2014. These major human epidemics of viruses that came from animal hosts were a sign. We should probably not be surprised that these signals of threat went unheeded. We are all guilty of confirmation bias – ignoring information that doesn't match our own view or experience of the world. How many of us have experienced a pandemic? Catastrophes reveal the weaknesses of human memory. How can one plan for a random rare event, even if it is certain to happen? Surely the sacrifices in the short term will be too great? But, as seismologist Lucy Jones argues in *The Big Ones* (2018), 'Natural hazards are inevitable; the disaster is not.'[17]

Risks can be measured and quantified. As Laurie Garrett and the Institute of Medicine showed so clearly, the dangers of a new epidemic have been known and understood since HIV emerged in the 1980s. And what about HIV? 75 million people have been infected with HIV since the start of that epidemic; 32 million people have died. HIV may not have swept through the world with the pace of SARS-CoV-2, but its shadow remains immeasurably greater and should have alerted governments to be ready for an outbreak of a new viral threat.

In times of crisis, public and politicians alike understandably turn to experts. On this occasion the experts – scientists who have modelled and simulated our possible futures – made assumptions that turned out to be mistaken. The UK imagined a pandemic in the image of influenza. The influenza virus is not benign. Annual deaths from influenza vary widely, with a recent peak in the UK of 28,330 deaths in 2014/15 and a low of 1,692 deaths in 2018/19. But influenza is not COVID-19.

China, by contrast, was scarred by its experience of SARS. When the government realised that a new SARS virus was circulating, Chinese officials didn't advise hand-washing, a better cough etiquette and the disposal of tissues. They locked down entire cities and turned off the economy. Gabriel Leung in Hong Kong calls this response 'East Asian exceptionalism'. The long history of epidemics originating in the region – Asian influenza in 1957, the Hong Kong influenza pandemic in 1968, a series of avian influenza outbreaks in the 1990s and early 2000s, and finally SARS and MERS – had acted as a kind of 'sociological imprinting' on the Asian mind. They were ready for COVID-19. But, as one former secretary of state for health in England put it to me, our scientists suffered from a 'cognitive bias' towards the milder threat of influenza.

Perhaps that is why the key government committee, the New and Emerging Respiratory Virus Threats Advisory Group (NERVTAG), concluded on 21 February, three weeks after WHO had declared a PHEIC, that, with one exception, they had no objection to Public Health England's 'moderate' risk assessment of the disease threat to the UK population. That was a genuinely fatal error of judgement.

This failure to escalate the risk assessment led to mortal delays in preparing the NHS for the coming wave of infection. The desperate pleas I received during March and April from frontline NHS staff are painful to read. 'Nursing burnout is at an all-time high and a lot of our heroic nursing staff are on the verge of emotional breakdown.' 'It is sickening that this is happening, and that somehow this country thinks it's okay to let some members of staff get sick, get ventilated, or die.' 'I feel like a soldier going to war without a gun.' 'It's suicide.'

The availability of and access to appropriate personal protective equipment was appallingly bad for many nurses and doctors during the first wave of the pandemic. Some hospital trusts planned well. But many, maybe most, were unable to provide the necessary safety equipment to their frontline teams.

At every press conference, the government spokesperson always included the same line – 'We have been following the medical and scientific advice.' It's a good line. And it's partly true. But government knew – Exercise Cygnus – that the NHS was unprepared. Government knew it had failed to build the necessary intensive-care surge capacity to meet the likely patient demand. As one doctor wrote to me: 'It seems that nobody wants to learn from the human tragedy that happened in Italy, China, Spain . . . This is really sad . . . Doctors and scientists who are not able to learn from one another.'

The scientists and physicians leading the response to the pandemic in the UK said that keeping deaths from COVID-19 to below 20,000 would be a 'good outcome'. That line was breached on 25 April, 'a very sad day for the nation'.

The official government narrative was that the UK's National Health Service had succeeded in coping with the epidemic. Yet that assessment was only true because thousands of planned appointments and elective procedures were cancelled to create the capacity for the succeeding wave of COVID-19 admissions. 33,000 beds were cleared of patients in England alone to provide the space to absorb the expected influx of patients with COVID-19.

Despite the very best efforts of health workers, the NHS certainly did not cope. It was unable to deliver the necessary surge capacity beyond its normal service provision; it failed to implement a test, trace and isolate policy until late in the outbreak, and even then ineffectually; it did not provide adequate supplies of personal protective equipment, leaving health workers on the frontline of the outbreak response vulnerable to infection; and the separation of social care from the NHS left older citizens unprotected in care homes. One result of the massive displacement of thousands of planned operations, procedures and appointments was the creation of a backlog of work that will only be completed well into 2021 and will only worsen pressures on already stressed hospitals, community and primary care services, and social care. When Jenny Harries, England's deputy chief medical officer, called the UK's state of preparedness an 'international exemplar', most observers were astonished. The UK's response had been slow, complacent and flat-footed. The country was glaringly unprepared.

*

COVID-19 has revealed the astonishing fragility of our societies, our shared vulnerability. It has revealed our inability to cooperate, to coordinate and to act together. Perhaps we cannot control the natural world after all. Perhaps we are not quite as dominant as we once thought. If COVID-19 eventually imbues human beings with some humility, then possibly we will, after all, be receptive to the lessons of this deadly virus. Or perhaps we will sink back into our culture of complacent Western exceptionalism and await the next plague that will surely arrive. To go by recent history, that moment will come sooner than we think.

Something went badly wrong in the way many countries handled COVID-19. In the UK, the government had the services of some of the most talented researchers in the world on which to draw. But somehow there was a collective failure to recognise the signals that Chinese and Italian scientists were sending. The UK had the opportunity and the time to learn from the experience of other countries. For reasons that remain not entirely clear, the UK missed those signals and missed those opportunities.

Perhaps it was the regime of science policymaking that had gone wrong. I believe two charges can be fairly made against the current regime with respect to its handling of this pandemic. First, that it was corrupted – the system resulted in an abuse of entrusted power. It was an abuse of power because the system of science policy formation failed to act on clear and unambiguous signals from China that culminated in a PHEIC from WHO on 30 January. When a PHEIC was called, government scientific advisory committees, such as NERVTAG, together with the chief medical officer and chief scientific advisor, should have urgently started asking questions. They should have contacted their counterparts in China and Hong Kong – Bin Cao, George Gao, George Leung – to seek first-hand testimony about what was happening. They should have called WHO's country office in Beijing to understand their assessment of the situation in Wuhan. If they had done so, our most senior scientific advisors would have heard the same messages so starkly reported in their published papers from January – a pandemic of a bitterly toxic virus was on its way to Europe. The fact that they apparently took none of these actions is what constitutes the abuse of entrusted power.

Second, that it was collusive – scientists and politicians agreed to act together in order to protect the government, to give the illusion that the UK was an 'international exemplar' in preparedness and made the right decisions at the right time, based upon the science. Every day, as the pandemic moved its venomous way through the population, a minister would deliver a press briefing to announce the daily toll of infection and death. He or she would be flanked by a government scientist or medical advisor. When advisors were asked questions, they would speak with one voice in support of government policy. They never deviated from the political scripts they were given. Why was no PPE reaching frontline health workers? Instead of saying honestly that the lessons of Exercise Cygnus had not been acted upon, the scientific or medical advisor would say the government was doing its best and that PPE was on its way, when clearly it was not. Why was testing capacity so poor? Instead of saying honestly that the government had ignored

WHO's recommendation to 'test, test, test', the advisor would say that testing wasn't appropriate for the UK. Why did the government stop reporting mortality figures for the UK and other countries in the middle of the first wave? Instead of saying honestly that the government found those figures politically embarrassing, the advisor would say that such comparisons were spurious and, anyway, they were available elsewhere. Advisors became the public relations wing of a government that had failed its people.

*

Is British science really so corrupted and collusive? Is there no alternative to this broken system of obsequious politico-scientific complicity? Yes, there is.

'Is the government's objective to suppress infection or to manage the infection?', asked Sir David King at the first press conference of the newly formed Independent Scientific Advisory Group for Emergencies (iSAGE), held in May. The UK now had two SAGEs. The officially constituted SAGE provides scientific advice to support government decision-making during emergencies. It had seen its reputation collapse during the previous three months. Partly, this loss of credibility arose out of the group's unwillingness to be transparent about its participants and its proceedings. At a moment of national emergency, SAGE's pervasive secrecy and deference to ministers simply became unacceptable. The public had a right to know the evidence on which advice was being made to government

– advice that was not only protecting lives but also destroying livelihoods. But the official SAGE luxuriated in elite insouciance. It displayed a very British characteristic: an arrogance that suggests the British possess inherent superiority over others. Rarely has a publicly constituted body been so out of touch with the public mood for accountability.

The Independent SAGE published its membership before holding its first meeting. Sir David King was himself once chief scientific advisor to the UK government, the position now occupied by Sir Patrick Vallance. But King had put together a more gender- and ethnically diverse scientific group than the official SAGE – which had the look of a white male club. The new and more independent version of SAGE was also broader in the range of science upon which it drew. Public health was at its core, but it also included experts on epidemic modelling, behavioural science and public policy.

This wider intellectual reach made the recommendations of iSAGE more relevant to the UK's predicament. The first meeting was broadcast on YouTube, giving the public full access to the difficult judgements needed to steer the country out of lockdown. It also displayed the challenges faced by political decision-makers who had to ensure the country was prepared should a second wave of the pandemic ensue.

The early recommendations from iSAGE focused on five additional areas beyond seeking clarification of the government's overall objective in managing the pandemic. First, how was the government planning to ensure financial security for the most marginalised groups in society, including black, Asian and minority ethnic populations (a group that suffered four times the mortality rate from COVID-19)? This virulent coronavirus had revealed, exploited and accentuated deep socio-economic and racial disparities in the UK. As Zubaida Haque noted, the existing 'economic safety net is not enough.' Haque is deputy director of the Runnymede Trust and an expert on race equality. The government had ignored those least able to protect themselves, she argued.

Second, community public health and primary care systems needed to be urgently strengthened. Allyson Pollock is a professor of public health at Newcastle University. She pointed out that community public health had been decimated during the past decade. Third, improved long-term planning was needed to meet the needs of those most at risk of infection – by increasing intensive-care capacity, for example. Fourth, policies were needed to control borders – at seaports, at airports and for train services to Europe.

And, finally, the emphasis on vaccines as a means to return life to some measure of normality needed to be tempered by accepting that no vaccine was a going to be a perfect solution to ending the pandemic. As emphasised by Deenan Pillay, professor of virology at University College London, even if a vaccine was made and manufactured by the end of 2020, it was unlikely to be completely safe and effective, and it would almost certainly not be taken up universally. Although his pessimistic prediction has not been fully borne out by events – vaccines with 90 per cent efficacy had been delivered by the end of 2020 – his broader point remains true: vaccines are an important instrument for epidemic control, but they will need to be supplemented by continuing behaviours that reduce the risks of virus transmission.

King's argument for setting up a rival body to SAGE was that ensuring public trust in the scientific advice given to government demanded that those giving advice should not be dependent on the government.[18] Too many members of the official SAGE were government employees. The official SAGE allowed the participation of the architect of Brexit, Dominic Cummings, who had been appointed by Prime Minister Boris Johnson as his chief political advisor. The official SAGE became impossibly compromised.

This first meeting of iSAGE set a new standard for science policymaking. The openness of the process, vigour of discussion, and identification of issues barely discussed by politicians injected much needed candour into public and political debates about COVID-19. It's hard to predict the longevity of this new group. It continued its work throughout 2020, delivering important recommendations about regional tiering, testing and schools. But its point was quickly made. On the same day it held its first meeting, the government for the first time published the names of members of the official SAGE.

*

Eventually, some senior scientists found the collusion between science and government impossible to bear. They broke ranks. Nobel laureate Sir Paul Nurse went on the BBC's *Today* radio programme on 22 May to argue that the government was on the 'back foot'. 'Maybe there's a strategy there, I don't see it,' he said. 'We are desperate for clear leadership at all levels.'

*

I sat with the director-general of the WHO in Geneva in February. He was in despair. Dr Tedros had been criticised for not calling a PHEIC sooner. But when he did so, and when he subsequently asked for the modest sum of $675 million to help WHO combat the growing global pandemic, countries ignored his pleas. Most countries eventually took the right actions to extinguish the first wave of this pandemic. But their governments lost valuable time. There were preventable deaths. And as the second and third waves of the pandemic surged, lessons were not learned. The system failed. When the cycles of suppression and rebound have finally been broken by a vaccine, when life returns to some measure of normality, difficult questions will have to be asked and answered. Because we can't afford to fail again. We may not have a second chance.

4

First Lines of Defence

An epidemic is a sudden disastrous event in the same way as a hurricane, an earthquake, or a flood. Such events reveal many facets of the societies with which they collide. The stress they cause tests social stability and cohesion.

Dorothy Porter, *Health, Civilization and the State* (1999)

Were the countries hit hardest by COVID-19 just unlucky? I don't believe that chance can completely exonerate governments from their responsibility. But there is a peculiarity about this coronavirus and the way it is transmitted that makes it especially difficult to control.

Influenza is a straightforward viral infection. Its spread is predictable and follows the reproduction number with helpful rigour. That is, the number of secondary infections can fairly reliably be predicted from an index case. But SARS-CoV-2 is not influenza. And it is frustratingly unpredictable. In technical language, this coronavirus has a higher degree of variance in its transmission than influenza. Put more directly, as many as 80 per cent of infections are transmitted by just 10 per cent of those infected. Large numbers of people infected go on to infect no one. The R number is not a reliable means for judging viral spread, which may come as a surprise given the almost obsessive reporting of R by governments and their scientific advisors. But the fact is that COVID-19 is subject to a phenomenon called overdispersion.

Overdispersion means that some individuals are superspreaders of viral infection. If an infected person is in the right place at the right time, he or she will turbocharge viral transmission. Evidence has accumulated that in poorly ventilated, crowded, indoor environments with prolonged contact with others, especially with loud talking or singing, the risk of infection multiplies dramatically. That means hospitals, restaurants, bars, weddings, church services, residential care homes, public transport, dormitories, gyms, and large multigenerational households are particularly dangerous venues for the spread of disease. A low R number does not rule out a superspreading event with a virus that displays overdispersion.

The relevance for public policy is important. Certain settings are higher risk than others. Broad society-wide interventions – lockdowns, partial lockdowns or tiered mandates – may not always be as effective as one hoped. If you want to manage the risk of infection, avoiding crowded places, closed spaces and close contact will go a long way to reducing your probability of acquiring COVID-19.

This is where chance may have played a part. If a country had a few early superspreading events, the infection may have taken hold quickly and accelerated out of control before even the most robust public health system could have noticed. We will never know if some countries were unlucky. Even if they were, lessons can be drawn from the way those countries responded.

*

What does it mean to possess a health service? At the very least, it represents the commitment of people living in a society (past and present) to the twin ideas of solidarity and collective action. By solidarity I mean the feelings of empathy and responsibility we all feel and owe towards one another. Solidarity stands in opposition to the principles of individualism and competition which so dominate and shape our lives in twenty-first-century capitalist, and even authoritarian, nation-states.

The existence of, public support for, and continuous development of a health system suggests that we are prepared to make personal material contributions (e.g., through taxation) to institutions that protect and strengthen the lives not only of ourselves but also of others in our society. That willingness to act on behalf of others is the second feature of a health system — our commitment to a belief in our interdependence and reciprocal responsibility towards one another and also to the collective action necessary to make those feelings real and tangible.

The whole basis of our society depends upon these two principles. COVID-19 has tested their resilience. So many people have died, so many families are in mourning, so many communities have been left scarred by disease. We have been shocked by the power of a virus to throw our societies into chaos, to deprive us of our lives and liberties, and to destroy economies. COVID-19 invites us, calls on us, requires us to rethink who we are and what we value.

One fundamental shift in our thinking surely has to be around the concept of our security. Ever since the birth of the nation-state, security has been viewed as the protection of national borders and of each country's political sovereignty. An infectious disease such as SARS-CoV-2 transcends states, borders and sovereignty. A virus is not amenable to passport controls or military defeat, despite the frequent invocation of the idea of an 'invisible enemy'. No person, no country, can survive in splendid isolation.

COVID-19 has taught us to reimagine security as being about people and communities across borders, about our survival, our livelihoods and our dignity. Disease is a threat to our human security, and pandemics are the most dangerous threats of all. Pandemics disrupt every part of our society, leaving us wounded and vulnerable. Protecting our security is not only about having strong military defences. Our security also depends on strong social institutions – and an effective health system is the most important defence we have to protect that security. Think of the security of your own family if you do not believe me.

The Chinese government was deeply traumatised by its experience of SARS in 2002–3. China's leaders felt the threat a virus posed to their political model. The acceptance by the Chinese people of a government that restricted political freedoms in return for annual double-digit economic growth was a particular kind of social contract that carried inherent risks. For, if economic growth was endangered, the social contract that enabled the Chinese Communist Party to rule unchallenged would be in danger too. Not since the events of Tiananmen Square on 4 June 1989 had the Chinese regime felt so vulnerable. They now understand that national security means health security. And so they were ready.

When SARS-CoV-2 emerged, the first reaction of local officials in Wuhan was to suppress the evidence for its existence. The life of Li Wenliang will forever stand as an example of a courageous commitment to warn his fellow citizens of the impending threat. But once authorities in Beijing – and especially those in the National Health Commission (China's Ministry of Health), the China Center for Disease Control and Prevention and the Chinese Academy of Medical Sciences – learned of what was taking place in Hubei Province, they recognised the threat. If the virus took hold, the government would simultaneously have to cut the lines of viral transmission and protect its health system from being overwhelmed. China's government achieved both objectives through a deceptively simple innovation – facility-based isolation, or the Fangcang shelter hospital.[1]

These vast temporary hospitals, rapidly built in existing sports stadiums and exhibition halls, were used to isolate patients with COVID-19 from their families and workplaces. They provided food and basic medical care, enabling ongoing illness among those admitted to be monitored carefully. If a patient deteriorated, they could be transferred to a hospital with proper intensive-care facilities.

The word 'Fangcang' sounds like 'Noah's Ark' in Chinese. In Wuhan, three of these shelter hospitals were constructed and were ready to accept up to 4,000 patients with mild to moderate disease by early February. A further thirteen similar shelter hospitals were opened in the succeeding weeks, providing 12,000 beds. As the epidemic came under control and subsided, the hospitals were decommissioned, the last being closed by mid-March.

Why admit patients with mild disease to a shelter hospital instead of insisting on home isolation? The reason lay in the way in which the virus was being transmitted. With workplaces and public venues closed, most infections were being spread within families. China grasped the idea of overdispersion early on. It was essential to remove anyone who fell ill from a place where further transmission could take place.

Shelter hospitals released pressure from existing healthcare facilities. The approximately 80 per cent of patients with mild to moderate disease could be managed effectively and efficiently in these temporary hospitals, receiving basic medical care and, where necessary, oxygen and intravenous fluids. A patient's temperature, respiratory rate, oxygen saturation and blood pressure were all carefully followed. Mobile diagnostic units gave additional access to imaging and laboratory services. Any worsening of a patient's condition could be detected early, allowing for rapid referral to a hospital with more specialist healthcare facilities.

The organisation of Fangcang shelter hospitals contributed quickly to reducing the reproduction rate, R, of SARS-CoV-2.

They undoubtedly saved lives. The hospitals were staffed with doctors and nurses mobilised from outside Wuhan. As a group of Chinese doctors involved in the organisation and delivery of care to patients with COVID-19 noted, 'By embracing Fangcang shelter hospitals, many countries and communities worldwide could boost their response to the current COVID-19 pandemic as well as future epidemics and disasters.'

Sadly, many countries afflicted by COVID-19 were unable to respond in such agile and creative ways. Western countries relied on advice to self-isolate if infected with coronavirus. But as the pandemic continued, as trust in governments eroded, and as fatigue set in, many, perhaps most, people did not adhere to the advice. Governments were reluctant to impose strict enforcement. The result was that Western nations were unable to quarantine those who became infected. They were unable to control the pandemic.

*

While the epicentre of the pandemic was Wuhan, the virus quickly spread to other Asian nations. Singapore confirmed its first imported case of COVID-19 on 23 January. Inbound flights to the city-state were banned. Several clusters of disease were identified and close contacts were quarantined. A 'circuit-breaker' lockdown was implemented in April and lasted until June. Although Singapore is widely thought to have had one of the most successful responses to COVID-19 – the number of deaths per 100,000 population was 0.5, exceedingly low – political leaders did make one disastrous oversight, again underlining the vulnerability of the most marginalised people in our societies: they ignored their migrant workers. Singapore has over 300,000 poorly paid foreign workers from mostly South-East Asian countries, such as India and Bangladesh. They live in crowded dormitories with few health protections. When the virus hit, they were utterly exposed. The result is that, of Singapore's 60,000 infections, over 90 per cent are among migrant health workers. The government's blindness to the inequality in its midst stained an otherwise exemplary response.

Hong Kong also followed WHO's recommendation to 'test, test, test'. Those who were found to be positive for coronavirus were quarantined in hospital. Contacts were traced and told to self-isolate. Borders were strictly controlled – anyone arriving from a country with cases of COVID-19 was required to go into quarantine for fourteen days. Quarantine facilities were expanded. Schools were closed and people were encouraged to work from home. No lockdown was formally imposed. Instead, the public voluntarily chose to alter their behaviour, avoid mass gatherings and wear face masks. Again, as a result of perspicacious government action, Hong Kong was able to keep its total number of COVID-19 deaths to just over one hundred. The lessons of SARS two decades earlier had been successfully learned.

The coronavirus arrived in Taiwan on 21 January. By the end of 2020, according to the Johns Hopkins Coronavirus Resource Center, there had been only 600 confirmed cases of infection and seven deaths, putting deaths per 100,000 at an astonishingly low figure – 0.03 (to give some measure of comparison, Belgium's deaths per 100,000 were 128). The Taiwanese government's response has therefore been widely and rightly praised. The government put the country on high alert in January as the first reports of COVID-19 began to emerge from the Chinese mainland. Those entering Taiwan were screened for infection. After 21 January, Taiwan suspended all air travel to China and quarantined anyone arriving from the mainland. Personal protective equipment was secured, physical distancing implemented, schools were closed, quarantine centres established and mask wearing on public transport was mandated. The government maintained its vigilance. As 2020 ended, Taiwan insisted that all travellers to the country must provide a negative COVID-19 test to the authorities within three days of arrival. Chen Chien-jen, Taiwan's vice-president, is an epidemiologist. His understanding of the threat of this SARS-like pandemic likely made a crucial difference to Taiwan's response. But, because the country's observer status at WHO meetings is blocked by the Chinese government in Beijing, the world will not have a full and complete opportunity to learn from Taiwan's success.

In South Korea, the epidemic took a strange turn. Between 19 January and 18 February, the country reported only thirty cases and no deaths. Patient 31 changed all that. Within ten days there were 2,300 cases. Patient 31 was a superspreader – a person who passes the virus to a far larger number of people than predicted by R_0. She had travelled from Wuhan to Seoul and Daegu, visited a hospital to be treated for a road traffic injury, attended church services (with 1,100 others at the Shincheonji Church of Jesus) and went to a hotel. The government's response was decisive and comprehensive. It had learned bitter lessons from an outbreak of MERS in 2015. A task force was appointed, including all government ministries and regional and city administrations. This emphasis on coordination and transparency worked. The lesson the government learned from MERS was the importance of testing and tracing, with rigorous self-isolation. They closed schools, but they didn't impose a lockdown. The first wave of the epidemic peaked on 29 February, but it came back with a vengeance in August and has continued to simmer. 'Our anti-coronavirus efforts are facing a crisis,' said Chung Sye-kyun, South Korea's prime minister, in November.

Japan's first case of COVID-19 was diagnosed on 16 January 2020 in a Japanese citizen returning from Wuhan. Then Prime Minister Shinzo Abe moved quickly to establish an Anti-Coronavirus National Task Force. Schools were closed in February. By April, the government had declared a state of emergency. The policy of containment, followed by prevention, treatment and mitigation, worked. Testing was expanded early on. Compliance, with guidance on hygiene, mask wearing, and physical distancing, was high. The result was that Japan recorded a very low death rate from COVID-19 – only 1.5 deaths per 100,000 people. And it did so without imposing the kind of punishing lockdowns seen across Europe. But one casualty of the pandemic was the 2020 Summer Olympics, now postponed until 2021.

New Zealand was an even more astonishing story of success. This country of 5 million citizens had suffered only two thousand cases of COVID-19 and twenty-five deaths by the end of 2020. Its death rate per 100,000 people was impressively low – 0.5. Prime Minister Jacinda Ardern reacted quickly and decisively after the first case was reported on 28 February, in a woman who had returned home from Iran via Indonesia. By 21 March, Ardern had raised the country's alert level and launched a national test, trace and isolate programme. By 23 March, the country had reported 102 cases. That was enough to trigger a lockdown. 'We only have 102 cases', said Ardern, 'but so did Italy once.' She went hard and early. Fifteen days after confirmation of the first case, she launched the rapid escalation of non-pharmaceutical interventions. She closed the country's borders. And she called a state of national emergency on 25 March. The epidemic peaked in early April, and by 15 May New Zealand was returning to a reasonably normal life. By 9 August, the country had gone one hundred days with no community transmission of SARS-CoV-2 – elimination of the virus had been achieved.[2] Clusters of cases have been reported since then, but judicious balancing of alert levels with economic liberties has enabled the country to navigate the pandemic successfully. An early, intense response enabled rapid easing while maintaining strict border controls. Ardern is one of the few political leaders to emerge from the COVID-19 with her reputation enhanced. She had good fortune on her side. New Zealand is a relatively isolated country with a low population density. But her clear, consistent and confident messaging to the public was a model of political choreography in a crisis. In October 2020, New Zealanders went to the polls in a general election. Ardern won with a landslide.

The first Australian cases of COVID-19 were reported in January 2020. The country's first death was on 1 March. By the end of the year, Australia had kept its number of deaths below a thousand, with a mortality rate of four deaths per 100,000 people – a result that was, if not quite as spectacularly successful as the Asian nations, still highly creditable. The government did well because they acted promptly, implementing 'slow the spread' policies in March. Lockdown restrictions were progressively put in place, schools were closed, and strict border control measures were introduced. By April, numbers of COVID-19 cases were falling. A second wave came in June and a second lockdown was imposed on Melbourne in July, which lasted 112 days. Victoria declared a disaster in August. This second wave proved much more deadly. Overall, Australia seemed to have emulated the successes of its neighbours. But, in one area, it was vulnerable. Over two-thirds of deaths have been in residential care homes (and mostly in the state of Victoria). The reasons are disputed, but the creation of a free market in social care in 1997, which deregulated the sector and turned it into a profitable business, certainly contributed. Standards of care fell. Infection control was poor. And staff were underqualified. The care of older people in Australia had become a multibillion dollar industry outsourced to the private sector. A Royal Commission into Aged Care Quality and Safety branded the care of older people in an era of COVID-19 as 'deplorable'.

*

When the virus arrived in Europe, several countries were simply overwhelmed. The first diagnosed person was an employee of an automobile supplier who visited the company's headquarters in Bavaria, Germany, from Shanghai, China, on 20 January 2020. She had been infected with SARS-CoV-2 in Shanghai (after her parents had visited from Wuhan) and transmitted the virus to a German man, who tested positive on 27 January. The virus also entered Europe via a second, independent route. Italy suffered nothing less than a humanitarian catastrophe after the first major outbreak took place in the Lombardy region towards the end of February.

Europe suffered and suffered badly. A comprehensive analysis of how European countries performed during the first wave of the pandemic has been completed by a team of scientists led by Majid Ezzati at Imperial College London.[3] Around 206,000 more people died during the first wave than would have been expected had the pandemic not taken place. Deaths were evenly distributed between men and women. Ezzati identified four groups of countries. The first group had the highest mortality toll, defined as deaths from all causes, not only from COVID-19. Measuring all-cause mortality is important because it takes account of deaths from conditions that may not have been appropriately treated because of disrupted health services. Undiagnosed cancers and untreated heart disease, for example, were common outcomes during the first wave. The group of countries with highest all-cause mortality consisted of Belgium,

Italy, Spain, England and Wales, and Scotland. England and Wales, Italy and Spain accounted for 28 per cent, 24 per cent and 22 per cent of these excess deaths, respectively. A second group of countries had a lower, although still quite high, level of overall death – France, the Netherlands and Sweden. A third category had still lower levels of mortality – Austria, Switzerland and Portugal. And a final group miraculously avoided any detectable rise in all-cause mortality – Bulgaria, Slovakia, Czechia, Hungary, Poland, Norway, Denmark and Finland. What accounts for these differences?

Ezzati and his colleagues argue that there are three elements to understanding why some countries did well while others failed so abjectly. One group of determinants of death is the baseline age and health of the population. COVID-19 kills those who are older, sicker and poorer. If a country's population is older and afflicted with more disease, especially high blood pressure, heart disease, obesity, diabetes and other chronic conditions, all-cause mortality will be higher, especially for those who endure social and material deprivation. This is the syndemic – a synthesis of epidemics – in action. But European countries do not display differences that can completely account for the wide variation in COVID-19 outcomes.

A further explanation might be the government's response to the pandemic. Indeed, the differences in policies taken towards COVID-19 go a long way to explain why Bulgaria did so much better than England and Wales. The timing and stringency of lockdown, together with the extent and effectiveness of the country's test, trace and isolate system, were crucial influences on final mortality. Simply put, those countries that acted faster, with tougher resolve, and with agility in mobilising testing capacity averted more deaths.

A third possible factor is the strength and resilience of the health, public health and social care systems. Austria, for example, had three times more hospital beds per head of population than England and Wales and so was much better able to absorb the shock of the pandemic. In England, the NHS effectively shut down in order to meet the expected demand from patients with COVID-19. Many people died as a result. As in Australia, care homes were a particular source of avoidable deaths in Spain, the United Kingdom, Belgium, Italy, France and Sweden. The preparedness of the health and social care systems also played an important part in shaping a country's success or failure in responding to the pandemic.

Spain imposed a full lockdown and a state of emergency on 14 March. But the health system was wholly unprepared, with daily deaths peaking at one point at over 700. Even on 8 March, the government allowed hundreds of thousands of people to take part in nationwide marches for International Women's Day. Health workers had poor access to personal protective equipment, leaving 50,000 infected by May. Ordinary healthcare was disrupted. And care homes became particular points of vulnerability.

In Madrid, a skating rink was commandeered as a temporary emergency morgue. On 9 April, Médecins Sans Frontières issued an urgent alert to the Spanish authorities, warning that older Spanish citizens were dying alone in residential care homes and hospitals without their families. As the epidemic ebbed, it became clear that the Spanish government had badly underestimated how fast the virus could spread and the seriousness of the disease it caused. The first COVID-19 case was reported in Spain on 31 January and the country's first death was on 13 February. And yet politicians, and even scientists, failed to respond to these early warnings.

As the summer saw Spain's death toll mount, so calls for a national inquiry grew louder. On the frontline of this call was a global health scientist and activist, Helena Legido-Quigley. In August, she brought together a distinguished group of Spanish medical scientists and former government advisors to demand an independent evaluation of Spain's COVID-19 response. She wanted an investigation into the decisions taken by the central government and the governments of Spain's seventeen autonomous communities. This was not about blame. Instead, the inquiry 'should identify areas where public health and the health and social care system need to be improved.' Prime Minister Pedro Sánchez ignored the invitation to learn lessons from his country's predicament. By October, he was forced to declare a state of emergency to keep Madrid in partial lockdown as cases soared out of control.

In France, the outbreak began in early February at about the same time as in South Korea. Jean-Paul Moatti, former director and president of the prestigious French National Research Institute for Sustainable Development, was highly critical of the French government's response. He wrote, 'a South Korean strategy of mass testing, contact tracing, and physical distancing was not adopted in France.' Instead, France imposed a lockdown on 17 March. The country didn't have the laboratory capacity for mass testing, and the government claimed mass testing was not needed anyway. They reversed that position at the end of March. President Macron had set up a COVID-19 Scientific Council on 10 March. Its members included medical experts from fields ranging from immunology to public health, from virology to epidemiology, and from infectious disease to intensive care. There were non-medical representatives from the public too. All advice given by the council was published. But although French authorities were able to control the first wave successfully, the country suffered a severe second wave later in the year, beginning in August. A second lockdown was imposed in October. By the end of 2020, France had suffered over 60,000 deaths from COVID-19, with ninety-five deaths per 100,000 population, one of the worst outcomes in Europe.

One peculiarity of the French predicament was a debate that raged about the use of hydroxychloroquine. In March, a Marseilles-based infectious diseases expert, Didier Raoult, claimed to possess the 'endgame' to solve the pandemic. Based on what most commentators believe is unreliable research, Raoult proposed a combination of hydroxychloroquine and azithromycin as a treatment for COVID-19. But, in June, a clinical trial from the UK showed that this medicine had no significant benefits in the management of patients with COVID-19. Raoult is now facing disciplinary hearings, accused of spreading false information.

The COVID-19 outbreak in Germany began with a Chinese woman travelling to Bavaria from Shanghai on 19 January, after having met her parents who had come from Wuhan. By 27 January, the first case of infection was confirmed. A month later, after travel to Wuhan had been restricted, the German government established a crisis management committee that produced a National Pandemic Plan. The number of cases continued to rise, reaching over 3,000 by 13 March. Restrictions were imposed the following week, with the closure of schools, clubs and bars. Borders were strengthened. The government banned events with fifty or more people. Churches and shops were next to be closed, on 16 March. On 18 March, Chancellor Angela Merkel said that COVID-19 was Germany's biggest challenge since the Second World War. A 'contact ban' was introduced. Numbers of infections continued to rise, but the pace of that rise began to stabilise. By 3 April, 1,100 Germans had died. By 11 April that figure had more than doubled, to 2,736 deaths. Yet, by 15 April, Merkel was ready to ease restrictions. Some shops and schools began partly to reopen. Germany seemed to have avoided the calamity suffered by its neighbours.

How did Germany escape the fate of the UK, Italy, Spain and France? Germany started testing, contact tracing and isolating infected patients early in February. The government recommended physical distancing and a fourteen-day quarantine period faster than most other countries. And Germany's well-funded health system had sufficient intensive-care capacity to cope. The chancellor, Angela Merkel, a scientist herself, delivered clear and precise public messages. The response was effectively coordinated by the much respected Robert Koch Institute. Lines of viral transmission were therefore cut quickly. The country's federal structure may have played a part too. The epidemic was managed locally in communities rather than exclusively from Berlin. Cities established their own testing centres, creating a network of 170 laboratories across the country. Despite these good reasons, Germany's relatively soft landing as it emerged from the pandemic still remains something of an enigma. Would the country be so well prepared and fortunate if and when a second wave of the virus arrives?

By the end of 2020, although Germany did experience a second wave demanding a 'wave break' or partial lockdown, the country can fairly claim to be the European nation that handled the pandemic most successfully. The country suffered 33,000 deaths, much fewer than its neighbours, France, Spain and the UK. But more impressively, the number of deaths per 100,000 was thirty-nine. Perhaps surprisingly, the public has been less admiring. Germany has seen widespread protests against the government's safety measures. An anti-vaccination movement is growing.

Sweden was another outlier, but for different reasons. Anders Tegnell, the country's state epidemiologist, has been accused of pursuing a policy of herd or community immunity, which led to over 400,000 cases of COVID-19 by the end of 2020. But that is neither fair nor entirely true. The first case of COVID-19 was diagnosed on 31 January, in a woman returning from Wuhan. Although no national lockdown has been introduced, Tegnell has issued a series of strong recommendations, which most people have complied with – limits on mass gatherings, closure of secondary schools and universities, working from home, avoiding unnecessary travel, and physical distancing. His focus was on individual responsibility rather than political instruction. It was a huge gamble and a backlash began to grow. Older citizens in social care were hit especially hard. By May, half of all COVID-19 deaths had taken place in residential homes. By the end of the year, Sweden had suffered over 8,000 deaths, with eighty-three deaths per 100,000 population (the comparable figures for Sweden's Scandinavian neighbours Norway and Denmark were eight and twenty-one, respectively). Sweden chose a different path to address the pandemic – gentle guidance over hard rules. Political libertarians in other countries praised Tegnell and used the Swedish approach to castigate their own lockdown-loving governments. But those who celebrated Sweden's supposed successes were premature. Towards the end of 2020, infection rates exceeded those in Spain and the UK. Hospitalisations and deaths rose. Herd immunity was not achieved. Voluntary lockdowns were imposed. The second wave proved devastating for the country. In a television address at the end of the year, Sweden's King Carl XVI Gustav concluded that his country's response had 'failed'. Prime Minister Stefan Löfven agreed: 'Of course, the fact that so many have died can't be considered as anything other than a failure.'

With over 10 million confirmed cases of COVID-19 at the beginning of 2021, India has also struggled to steer a safe course through the pandemic. The country's first case was reported on 30 January. The government closed its international borders early, and a subsequent lockdown, the largest in the world, was praised by WHO as 'tough and timely'. Lockdown also gave the government time to prepare for the possible surge in cases. Still, India's diverse population, its harsh health inequalities, widening economic and social disparities, and distinct cultural features presented extreme challenges.

Although it is one country, India is in truth a nation of nations – twenty-eight quasi-autonomous states and eight union territories. Important and often impressive differences in preparedness and response emerged at state level. In Kerala, for example, state authorities drew on their experience with an outbreak of Nipah virus in 2018 to use extensive testing, contact tracing and community mobilisation to contain the virus and maintain a low mortality rate. Odisha's exposure to previous natural disasters meant crisis preparations were already in place and were simply repurposed to address COVID-19. Hospitals dedicated to admitting patients were quickly requisitioned. Maharashtra, which endured the highest number of diagnosed cases, used drones to monitor physical distancing during lockdown and applied a cluster containment strategy to control the disease within a defined geographic area. On identifying three or more COVID-19-positive patients, a 3 kilometre radius around a patient's home was surveyed house to house for fourteen days to detect further cases, contact trace and raise public awareness.

Rajasthan imposed curfews and a ban on spitting. Uttar Pradesh, India's most populous state, expanded its laboratory testing capacity. But, given the country's overall limited testing capacity, a sparse public health workforce and certain challenging disease characteristics, including mild and asymptomatic cases and rapid spread, it is unlikely that states were able to reach the levels of operational excellence needed to control the outbreak fully. Nevertheless, there was an extraordinary response from sections of civil society. To fight fake news about the pandemic, the Indian Scientists' Response to COVID-19 became a grass-roots initiative to neutralise disinformation. States deserve much of the credit for the country's partly successful response. There were important lessons for other countries to learn from India.

One shortcoming of India's COVID-19 response was the low rate of testing. Another constraint was an acute shortage of health workers, while yet another consisted of the large communities living in slums with no possibility for physical distancing. The government's sudden enforcement of lockdown also disadvantaged already vulnerable populations. There was a mass exodus of migrant workers, and concerns rose about starvation among those who worked in the informal economy. Implementing public health measures is always difficult in places with overcrowded living conditions and inadequate hygiene and sanitation. Non-COVID-19 health services have been disrupted. The pandemic was also used to fan anti-Muslim sentiment and violence after a gathering linked to the group Tablighi Jamaat was identified as the source of a large cluster of cases. Yet India's relatively young population – two-thirds are under thirty-five years of age – may well have protected the country from a much more severe health crisis.

As for the US, pictures of makeshift mass graves in New

York state being dug and filled with wooden coffins taken from refrigerated trucks by prisoners wearing hazmat suits perhaps best summed up the lamentable response by President Trump's administration. His suggestion that patients with COVID-19 might benefit from injections of disinfectant, made at a press conference on 24 April, defined the farce that the American political response became. By May, President Trump was describing the 'attack' of COVID-19 as being worse than Pearl Harbor and 9/11. The US response has been as pitiful as it has been surprising. Opinion polls put only Boris Johnson and Xi Jinping below President Trump in terms of public trust. A superpower – or its reputation at least – had been slain by a virus.

Elsewhere, there was chaos. Brazil's President Jair Bolsonaro responded to a question about rapidly rising numbers of COVID-19 cases by saying, 'So what? What do you want me to do?' In Russia, President Putin faced an economic crisis that threatened the stability of his government. He was forced to cancel 9 May Victory Day celebrations that would have triumphantly marked his amendment to the constitution designed to keep him in office until 2036.

*

One important consequence of the COVID-19 health emergency was the focus it put on the most vulnerable individuals and communities in our society. In the UK, for example, 1.3 million people were 'shielded' during the first wave of the pandemic. This group included those who had undergone an organ transplant, patients with specific types of cancer and who were undergoing treatment with chemotherapy or radiotherapy, people with severe respiratory disease, those with rarer diseases who were more at risk from infection, and women who were pregnant. They were advised to stay isolated and avoid any face-to-face contact for at least three months.

But just who should be defined as 'vulnerable'? Some critics argued that the definition of those at risk should have been far more capacious. It was known, for example, that older patients had a higher risk of complications and death from COVID-19. Across the UK population, there were 5.7 million people over the age of seventy. Surely they were vulnerable too. The epidemiology of deaths from COVID-19 also showed a clear relation between having an underlying health condition and death. An additional 2.7 million people under the age of seventy lived with a condition such as heart disease or diabetes. The total number of vulnerable people in the UK was therefore much higher – 8.4 million people.[4] And what about those who were living in care homes, the homeless, those in prison, or people who lived with severe mental health problems? They were excluded from the government's gaze.

If the NHS has faced its most serious emergency since it was founded in 1948, then the social care system underwent nothing less than devastation – which took place without any politician seeming to know or understand what was happening. But by the end of April the scale of the social care tragedy had become all too clear.

On 28 April, the Office for National Statistics reported that, up to 17 April, 2,906 people had died in care homes from COVID-19-related causes. Additional data showed that, between 18 and 24 April, there had been a further 2,375 COVID-related deaths in social care settings. In total, from 10 to 24 April, 4,343 people had died in residential care and nursing homes from the direct effects of the pandemic. Whereas hospital deaths peaked around 10 April and were now seeing a slow decline, the epidemic raging through care homes was only just beginning. One of the lasting legacies of COVID-19 will be the silent human destruction it wreaked on the most unprotected older members of society.

Black and Asian men and women were four times more likely to die from COVID-19 compared with their white counterparts. This additional risk in particular ethnic communities intersected with pre-existing inequalities in society. After taking account of age and other socio-economic characteristics, the risk of a COVID-19-related death for men and women of black ethnicity reduced to two times more likely than among those of white ethnicity. The Office for National Statistics concluded that 'the difference between ethnic groups in COVID-19 mortality is partly a result of socio-economic disadvantage and other circumstances, but a remaining part of the difference has not yet been explained.' Almost two-thirds of health workers who have died were from an ethnic minority. The UK government has established an inquiry to understand why black, Asian and minority ethnic communities are in special jeopardy.

Every government that put its population into lockdown adopted a similar message – stay at home. But that message may have backfired. People did stay at home, even when they had symptoms of life-threatening illness, such as a heart attack, stroke or cancer. The true toll of death from the pandemic will have to include those who didn't receive the emergency care they so urgently needed. The shadow of the pandemic on society will be long and dark.

Health workers were shockingly unprotected. No other group in society was at more immediate risk than those whose job it was to care for people with COVID-19. And yet in many countries they were the least protected. WHO had recommended high standards for the personal protective equipment that should have been available to health workers – a full body gown, a fit-tested mask and visor, and rubber gloves. And yet in many countries all that was available were thin plastic aprons that left arms and legs exposed, inadequate surgical masks, and rubber gloves that left arms vulnerable.

Health workers were left unprotected because governments had failed to procure sufficient supplies of protective equipment as soon as a PHEIC had been declared. It was a stunning act of administrative omission and certainly cost the lives of dozens of health workers in some of the most affected countries. At daily 10 Downing Street press briefings, government ministers would claim that personal protective equipment was being delivered to the frontlines of care and that health workers were safe. At best, these statements turned out to be overpromises. At worst, they were bare-faced lies.

As the epidemic in the UK took hold during March, I received hundreds of messages from health workers on the frontlines of care in the NHS, a collective cry of anguish about their abandonment by government. Their testimonies should be read and remembered: our government deserted the nation's most precious line of human defence.

'It's terrifying for staff at the moment. Still no access to PPE [personal protective equipment] or testing.'

'The situation is horrendous for everyone.'

'There's been no guidelines, it's chaos.'

'I don't feel safe. I don't feel protected.'

'We are literally making this up as we go along.'

'It feels as if we are actively harming patients.'

'We need protection.'

'Total carnage.'

'Humanitarian crisis.'

'Forget lockdown. We are going into meltdown at many practices.'

'The hospitals in London are overwhelmed.'

'The public and media are not aware that today we no longer live in a city with a properly functioning Western healthcare system.'

'How will we protect our patients and staff? I am speechless. It is utterly unconscionable. How can we do this? It is criminal. We feel completely helpless.'

'Brutal on the ground.'

'The tsunami is coming.'

'The situation is dire.'

'It is a national scandal.'

'There is serious failure of leadership.'

'There is a huge staffing crisis.'

'WHO PPE standards are not followed.'

'When generals have lost wars (lives) they have been tried for treason. What is the appropriate response in our circumstances?'

'We feel completely abandoned.'

'We feel it's a completely negligent approach and not safe at all.'

'I can't tell you how distraught we feel. It's beyond words.'

'Is anybody actually listening to the concerns and acting?'

'We have been so disappointed with the UK's late response.'

'This is playing with lives.'

'Inadequate PPE, no scrubs, not testing staff.'

'Totally inadequate PPE. No N95 masks. Being sent like lambs to the slaughter.'

'Today was shambolic in terms of PPE.'

'Sleepwalking into this totally unequipped and unprepared when we had the luxury of two months to prepare.'

'Patients are now dying of perfectly treatable conditions.'

'Seeing patients with no gowns or goggles.'

'It seems that nobody wants to learn from the human tragedy that happened in Italy, China, Spain.'

'Ongoing rationing and denying staff access to PPE.'

'Things on the frontline are getting worse, not better.'

'There is a huge mismatch about how the situation is presented publicly and the reality.'

'Colleagues have to attend disciplinary meetings for speaking out . . . I never thought I lived in a country where freedom of speech is discouraged.'

*

During the pandemic, UK government ministers encouraged the public to stand outside their homes every Thursday evening at 8 pm to 'clap for carers'. This display of support for frontline health workers was a moving mass public tribute to those who were risking and sacrificing their lives every day in settings of acute danger. But the government's injunction to celebrate carers was tinged with hypocrisy.

One doctor who died on the frontlines of COVID-19 care was Dr Abdul Mabud Chowdhury. He was a 53-year-old consultant urologist who worked at the Homerton Hospital in London. He had appealed to the government for 'appropriate PPE' to 'protect ourselves and our families', and he died of COVID-19 at the peak of the epidemic in London. His son, Intisar Chowdhury, has asked the government for a public apology for its failures to protect health workers from infection. So far, the government has provided no such apology. The closest it came was a comment by the home secretary, Priti Patel: 'Sorry to anyone who feels they had not had enough protection.' Intisar Chowdhury spoke for many health workers when he pointed out that 'Priti Patel's apology is not a real apology.'

*

Western countries spend a large proportion of their wealth on health. They have highly sophisticated health systems. And they have an extremely well-educated health workforce. One might wonder why the medical leaders in these countries did not do more to alert their governments in January to the impending catastrophe that was about to befall their populations.

In the UK, we have the medical Royal Colleges, the Academy of Medical Sciences, the British Medical Association, Public Health England, the Faculty of Public Health and an array of health think tanks, such as the King's Fund and Nuffield Trust. Yet none reinforced the urgent call to action in early February after WHO declared a PHEIC. That declaration fell on deaf ears within what one might call Britain's 'medical establishment'. Why?

I don't have an answer to this question. I don't believe there was a conspiracy of silence. But there was silence nonetheless. Perhaps the leaders of these bodies, all distinguished scientists and physicians, didn't read the reports coming out of China. Or perhaps they did but didn't appreciate their importance. Perhaps they didn't understand what a PHEIC meant. Perhaps they understood exactly what was happening but didn't want to criticise government publicly for fear of losing their seat of influence at the political table.

Whatever the reasons, the leadership of medicine in the UK and in many other Western nations let down those they were supposed to protect. They let down the old, the sick and the vulnerable. They betrayed the very people who had invested their trust – and their taxes – in modern medicine. It was a grubby betrayal, a stain on the leadership of a profession whose frontline workers had given so much.

Part of the answer to these systemic failures may lie in a new idea to enter the lexicon of health – the resilient health system. After the West African Ebola virus disease outbreak of 2015, politicians and policymakers understood the need to build health services that could absorb, withstand and learn from external shocks while retaining their fundamental functions and adapting and transforming to soften the impacts of future shocks. The idea of resilience is still only that – an idea. What does a resilient health system or resilient health service mean in practice? There are some obvious headline elements: adequate financing; a sufficiently large and skilled health workforce; accurate information to guide a response; transparent and accountable leadership; good supplies of essential medicines and health technologies; and the surge capacity to provide additional health services when needed while maintaining everyday clinical care.

One lesson of COVID-19 is that every country must now begin a national conversation about how far it is willing to go – and how much the public is willing to pay – for a health system that can save lives when a pandemic arrives again. As it surely will.

5

The Politics of COVID-19

... health professionals of the 21st century will find that they have entered what must become politicised professions. There is nowhere else to go.

Julian Tudor Hart, *The Political Economy of Health Care* (2006)

The response of governments to COVID-19 represents the greatest political failure of Western democracies since the Second World War. A government's first responsibility is its duty of care to citizens. Early government inaction led to the avoidable deaths of thousands of those citizens.

The failures were legion. First, there was a failure of technical advice. Despite possessing some of the world's most talented scientists, nations such as the US, Italy, Spain, France and the UK were unable to harness their knowledge and skills to deliver timely recommendations to forestall the terrifying human impacts of the pandemic.

Partly, this failure was because of a cognitive bias. The expectation in the Western world was that the next infectious pandemic was likely to be a new strain of influenza. The idea that a more severe SARS-like virus might strike was not taken seriously. The relatively small number of scientists advising governments existed in groups that did not explicitly consider alternatives to their dominant expectation – they suffered from a disabling 'group think'. Did those scientists read and take seriously the early reports of COVID-19 coming from China, reports that clearly and unambiguously warned of the clinical severity and pandemic potential of the new virus? Did they seek guidance from doctors and scientists in countries that first experienced the effects of COVID-19? If not, why not?

Second, there was a failure of the political process after receiving advice from scientists. During the outbreak, governments repeatedly claimed they were 'following the science'. But the task of politicians is not merely to accept the scientific advice they are given. They have an obligation to probe, to analyse and to question. Scientists advise, ministers decide. By not questioning the advice they received, or at least by not questioning it to any significant degree, politicians allowed themselves to believe that the pandemic could be withstood and contained without more urgent action.

Third, there were egregious failures of political leadership. Countries failed to establish teams that could develop a vision and a set of values for managing the pandemic. They failed to build trust and confidence among their publics. They failed to act decisively. And they failed to listen, to show humility and to learn from failure. Indeed, many governments actively resisted efforts to learn lessons or even denied that there were lessons to learn.

Fourth, there were catastrophic failures of preparedness. Despite the evidence from Wuhan, political leaders failed to acquire the necessary supplies of personal protective equipment, failed to construct necessary surge diagnostic and clinical capacities, and failed to protect other health services so that usual care could still be offered to those who needed it.

Fifth, there were failures of implementation. Countries often could not expand services to the scale needed in the time available. From testing and tracing to access to ventilators, political leaders struggled to keep ahead of the advancing first and then second and third waves of viral infection. This failure left them unable to manage the response to COVID-19 effectively as the pandemic evolved. It left them unable to plan properly for their lockdown exit strategies.

And, finally, there were serious failures of communication. The messages delivered to the public were often too little, too late. Advice was sometimes confused, contradictory or just plain misleading. U turns became the norm. When President Trump mused about the possible efficacy of ultraviolet light and disinfectants for preventing and treating COVID-19, he displayed astonishing irresponsibility at a time of national emergency.

Together, these failures constituted an extreme example of state negligence – a failure of governments to exercise their duty of care by ignoring evidence of possible danger, thereby exposing people to the risk of severe, sometimes fatal, harm. The evidence shows that governments could reasonably have been expected to know the risks posed by this new virus. They could reasonably have been expected to implement precautions to have diminished those risks. It was within the power of governments to have prevented this human crisis. They failed to prevent. They omitted to save. Their peoples were abandoned at a moment of spectacular vulnerability. Governments were causally complicit and responsible for these failures.

This message of gross incompetence is not welcome in Western political, medical or even media circles. It conflicts with a geopolitical narrative that casts China as a negative and destructive influence in international affairs. Instead, the preference has been to blame China and WHO. The claim is that China hid the fact of COVID-19. The claim is that WHO colluded with China in a cover-up of enormous proportions.

In April, President Trump initiated 'serious investigations' into China's handling of the COVID-19 outbreak. 'We are not happy with China,' he said on 27 April. 'We believe [the virus] could have been stopped at the source and it wouldn't have spread all over the world.' He called on the Chinese government to be held accountable for its errors, and he threatened to seek financial compensation from Beijing.

There are many reasons to be critical of contemporary China – repression of free speech; imprisonment of dissidents; human rights abuses in Tibet and Xinjiang. But one should perhaps try to put oneself in the position of Chinese policymakers. The common Western narrative about China is that, as the country's economy has grown, so have its strategic political, economic and military ambitions. China, led by an authoritarian Chinese Communist Party, now represents a threat to Western leadership in the free world. The evidence is surely all too clear – China's Belt and Road Initiative, its increasingly aggressive stance towards Hong Kong and Taiwan, and its claims over islands in the South China Sea. China has to be contained.

The Chinese perspective is very different. After a century of humiliation at the hands of a colonially minded West, China, proud of its 5,000-year-old civilisation, finally achieved independence in 1949. The country grew erratically and with terrifying mistakes under Mao Zedong, but he at least succeeded in establishing secure national borders. Deng Xiaoping created the conditions for economic expansion, lifting as many as 800 million people out of poverty. The task for every Chinese leader since has been to protect the territorial independence and integrity won by Mao and the economic security achieved by Deng. As China advances, so there is more and more material success to protect. Many of China's policymakers will argue that the government's actions should be seen not as aggressive, but as defensive.

In the case of COVID-19, China's scientists and physicians acted decisively and responsibly to protect the health of the Chinese people within this historical context. They warned their government, their government alerted WHO (albeit indirectly), and WHO warned the world. Western democracies failed to listen to those warnings. There are questions for both the Chinese government and WHO to answer. But to blame China and WHO for this global pandemic is to rewrite the history of COVID-19 and to marginalise the failings of Western nations.

*

It is understandable that Western countries would prefer to diminish their own responsibilities. Their governments are facing difficult questions about what they knew and when they knew it. And they are facing their own crises of trust. Polling during the outbreaks consistently showed disapproval over the responses of Western governments. At the peak of the first wave of the epidemic in the UK, for example, polls showed disapproval rates rising and a fall in confidence that the government had acted quickly enough. The rejection of President Trump in the US election in November 2020 was the most powerful example of that loss of public trust. Governments needed a new line of defence. And attack, they believed, was their best form of defence.

Placing responsibility for the pandemic on a country already distrusted by many citizens and an international agency that most people had barely heard of were easy diversions. And it seemed to work. Anti-China sentiment grew. And, although WHO received support from many European capitals after President Trump's decision to withdraw funding from the agency, there was little direct opposition to the US government's aggressive stance. After the SARS outbreak in 2002–3, WHO's prestige and influence had never been greater. After COVID-19, its reputation had never been in more jeopardy. The arrival of President Biden to the White House offers an opportunity for a global reset in relations with WHO and a re-engagement of the US in global coordination of the pandemic response.

Multilateralism was once again the victim, bloodied and wounded in a geopolitical war of words. Great power rivalry was ushering in a second Cold War, which dominated and shaped the international response to COVID-19. Globalism, international solidarity and cooperation between states were sacrificed in favour of unilateralism, nationalism and populist self-interest. It was a sad and disappointing contrast to the unanimity among nations following the SARS outbreak in 2002–3. The war against WHO was an unexpected twist in the story of COVID-19. As the world's only global health agency, WHO tries hard to be strictly apolitical, often to the frustration of its partners and supporters in civil society who want it to flex its political muscles more readily. Its dependency on budget contributions from its member states means that the agency is exquisitely sensitive to criticism from those same member states. To retain continued financial backing, each director-general must work hard to keep its richest donors happy.

When I first began visiting WHO's headquarters in Geneva in the 1990s, senior officials repeatedly reminded me that a quarter of their budget came from the US government. Whatever WHO said or did always had to be reflected through the prism of US interests. And yet during COVID-19, and despite close collaboration between WHO scientists and technical specialists at the CDC in Atlanta, WHO became one of the chief targets of the US administration. The attack by President Trump, accusing the organisation of being 'China-centric', became an unrivalled moment of vulnerability in the agency's 72-year history.

Dr Tedros sought to fight back, as diplomatically as he could –

The United States of America has been a longstanding and generous friend to WHO, and we hope it will continue to be so. We regret the decision of the President of the United States to order a halt in funding to the World Health Organization. With support from the people and government of the United States, WHO works to improve the health of many of the world's poorest and most vulnerable people . . . WHO is reviewing the impact on our work of any withdrawal of US funding and we will work with our partners to fill any financial gaps we face and to ensure our work continues uninterrupted.

But the political rift was deep, the partnership broken. Republican congressional members backed President Trump. The chairman of the Senate Finance Committee, Chuck Grassley, accused WHO of being 'slow to raise the global alarm' about the new coronavirus. In a letter to Dr Tedros, Grassley wrote that, 'Unfortunately, there is ample reason to question WHO's response to early signs of this outbreak in China. The lack of independent analysis and advice in the face of initial misleading public messaging from China has resulted in several countries scrambling to make up for lost time.'

When challenged about his decision, President Trump doubled down: 'They called it wrong. They call it wrong. They really, they missed the call.' A group of congressional

Republicans signed a letter calling on Dr Tedros to resign before US funding was restored.

All who know WHO understand that the agency is an imperfect institution. It is a bureaucracy that puts process before action, diplomacy before advocacy, and compromise before perseverance. WHO is a creature of its member states, reflecting their weaknesses, defects and frailties. Every new director-general pledges to reform WHO, and every director-general stumbles amid its glutinous protocols. But WHO serves a vital role. It gathers the world's best scientists to set standards for health, standards that countries use to advance the wellbeing of their peoples. In the poorest nations of the world, WHO provides indispensable support to ministries of health, health services and health workers.

The world needs a strong WHO to protect the human and health security of the world's poorest peoples, and the world needs a strong US government to support WHO both financially and politically. The sudden collapse of US backing for the organisation was a severe setback for global health security. The relationship between WHO and the US government could not be healed while both Dr Tedros and President Trump remained in their positions. One or both would have had to depart their roles before relations could be restored. The election of President Biden offers a moment for hope. His appointment in November 2020 of a thirteen-member Transition COVID-19 Advisory Board, drawing on internationally recognised and respected figures such as Eric Goosby, who had served as the US global AIDS coordinator and is currently the UN special envoy on tuberculosis, signalled a return of the US to the global family of nations struggling to control the pandemic.

*

I have already discussed the many strange stories of disinformation – the infodemic – that emerged during the crisis of COVID-19. What was even more surprising and unexpected was that governments themselves resorted to political disinformation campaigns in order to defend their own roles in managing the outbreak. These efforts to rewrite the narrative of COVID-19 are important to document. Just as there has been a struggle to contain the outbreak, so there is a struggle to control the way the public views government management of the outbreak.

In the UK, for example, ministers have claimed they did not pursue a policy of herd immunity early in the epidemic. The statements from politicians and science advisors clearly prove the opposite. Ministers argue that they have always supported testing for the virus. On the contrary, Jenny Harries, the deputy chief medical officer, made clear that testing was not appropriate for the UK. Ministers say that they have always prioritised the protection of older people living in care homes. The figures for deaths in care homes in several European countries show otherwise. The constantly repeated message of 'stay at home – protect the NHS – save lives' suggested that protecting the public has been the overriding objective of the UK government.

In fact, that message became official government policy only when Prime Minister Boris Johnson spoke to the nation on 23 March instructing people to stay at home. And then there was the statement that the UK was an 'international exemplar' in pandemic preparedness. The numbing toll of deaths displays the complete deceit of that claim.

I became entangled in one effort to manipulate the government's message to its advantage. On 19 April, the *Sunday Times* Insight team published a detailed analysis entitled, 'Coronavirus: 38 days when Britain sleepwalked into disaster'. The central thesis of the article was one that I had articulated in evidence to the House of Commons Select Committee on Science and Technology on 25 March – namely, that the government had wasted February and early March when it should have prepared for the arrival of the pandemic into the UK. The *Sunday Times* wrote, 'The government ignored warnings from scientists and lost a crucial five weeks in the fight to tackle the coronavirus, despite being in a perilously poor state of preparation for a pandemic.'

That same weekend, the government put out a long rebuttal, in which they wrote:

The editor of the Lancet, on exactly the same day – 23 January – called for 'caution' and accused the media of 'escalating anxiety' by talking of a 'killer virus' and 'growing fears'. He wrote: 'In truth, from what we currently know, 2019-nCoV has moderate transmissibility and relatively low pathogenicity. There is no reason to foster panic with exaggerated language.' The Sunday Times is suggesting that there was a scientific consensus around the fact that this was going to be a pandemic – that is plainly untrue.

This government statement was an extraordinary twisting of the truth, Kremlinesque in its audacity. My tweet, sent on 24 January, was commenting on lurid newspaper headlines that did indeed risk fostering panic. Panic is never a good public health strategy. Instead, what was needed was a careful and thoughtful discussion of the evidence from China and what it meant for the UK.

Later that same day, 24 January, I tweeted a link to the first paper *The Lancet* published describing the seriousness of the clinical presentation of COVID-19. I sent a second tweet with a link to a second paper published that day proving person-to-person transmission. In a further tweet I called what was taking place in Wuhan 'A novel coronavirus outbreak of global health concern'. The next day, 25 January, I drew attention to the issue of intensive-care capacity and asked why there had as yet been no discussion of what was clearly an urgent clinical challenge: 'A third of patients so far have required admission to ICU . . . Few countries have the clinical capacity to handle this volume of acutely ill patients. Yet no discussion.'

On 26 January, I tweeted, 'It's now imperative to recall WHO's IHR Emergency Committee to review once again the evidence for and against declaring a Public Health Emergency of International Concern. The needle is moving towards the affirmative.' On 30 January, the director-general of WHO did indeed declare a PHEIC. The facts were utterly opposite to the message from 10 Downing Street. There was an international scientific consensus. The government had simply chosen to ignore it.

In Jacques Ellul's study of the techniques used to manipulate the truth, *Propaganda*, he writes, 'Extreme propaganda must win over the adversary and at least use him by integrating him into its own frame of reference.'[1] The machine of government disinformation was perfectly proving Ellul's disturbing observation. On 10 May, Prime Minister Boris Johnson spoke to the nation. He said of COVID-19, 'We didn't fully understand its effects.' His plaintive excuse will likely become the core defence of his government in the subsequent public inquiry into why the UK failed so conspicuously to protect its citizens. It is a defence that can be and must be refuted.

*

COVID-19 is not a crisis about health. It is something much worse.

Every evening during the peak of the first wave of the pandemic in the UK, citizens could scour graphs presented by medical and scientific advisors at a daily government press briefing. Was the pandemic advancing or in retreat? New cases of COVID-19. People in hospital with COVID-19. Critical care beds with COVID-19 patients. Daily COVID-19 deaths in hospital. And then the final and bluntly worded 'global death comparison' – a graph that government scientists actively or passively censored in May as mounting mortality began to embarrass their hitherto crass confidence.

Those with responsibility for leading us through this emergency have called it 'a once in a century global health crisis'. This statement is incorrect on at least two grounds. First, because we cannot know what the rest of the century will bring. It is highly probable that the pandemic of SARS-CoV-2 will be neither the last nor the worst global health crisis of the present century. But, second, and more importantly, this global calamity is not a crisis concerning health. It is a crisis about life itself. We have been tempted in recent years to assume the omnipotence of our species. The idea of the Anthropocene places human activity as the dominant influence on the future for life on our planet. Although this newest of geological eras is supposed to underline the harm our species is doing to fragile planetary systems, paradoxically it also asserts our supremacy. SARS-CoV-2 has revealed the hubris of this view. Our species has many reasons to be self-critical about the effects of our way of life on planetary sustainability. But we are only one species among many, and we are certainly not a dominant influence when faced with a virus that can destroy life with such ease and facility.

If this pandemic is a crisis about life itself, what tentative conclusions might we draw from the effects of COVID-19 so far on human society?

Some clues will be found in the work of Didier Fassin, who studied medicine in Paris before turning to public health and anthropology. Fassin's starting point is the awareness we must all have for the unequal lives we see around us every day. That observation must surely invite us to reflect on the value our society attaches to each human life. We live in a moral economy as well as a market economy. That moral economy is concerned with 'the production, circulation, appropriation, and contestation of values as well as affects around . . . life'.[2] What are those values?

In trying to answer that question we somehow have to reconcile 'life as a fact of nature and as a fact of experience'. We can view COVID-19 as a biological challenge to understand, treat and prevent. But we should also understand it as a biographical event in the lives of millions of people. And this is where disease makes its entrance. 'Sickness', Fassin writes, 'sits at the meeting point of biology and biography.' Fassin divides his inquiry into inequality into three parts.

First, he identifies forms of life, by which he means 'ways of being in the world'. The daily insecurities faced by so many citizens draw attention to 'the predicament of contemporary democracies, incapable of living up to the principles that constitute the foundation of their very existence.' The vulnerabilities and precariousness of lives are both universal facts and particular experiences.

Second, he points to an ethics of life. He contrasts the rising legitimacy of those who have a biologically defined and 'empirically robust' proof of disease with the declining legitimacy of lives lived in a particular social setting (such as one of poverty). The physical has prevailed over the political. Fassin calls this ethical trend one of 'biolegitimacy' – a legitimacy of life defined only in biological terms. Life is reduced purely to its physical expression. There is no room for understanding the political conditions within which a life exists. There is no possibility of mobilising public sentiment to defend threats to political lives – lives marked, for example, by inequality. The physical life is legitimate. The political life is not. SARS-CoV-2 preferentially afflicts those who are more vulnerable, less well rewarded and more invisible to those with power.

Third, Fassin focuses on the politics of life, the government of populations, and the effects of politics on human lives. He is interested in how the actions of political regimes differentially influence human lives and reinforce the unequal worth of some of those lives in society. The 'politics of life', he writes, 'are always politics of inequality.'

So what must we say about the politics of COVID-19? We must say, I think, that it is our task to uncover the biographies of those who have lived and died with COVID-19. It is our task to resist the biologicalisation of this disease and instead to insist on a social and political critique. It is our task to understand what this disease means to the lives of those it has afflicted and to use that understanding not only to change our perspective on the world but also to change the world itself. As Fassin himself concludes, our 'critique does not have to choose between militancy and lucidity.'

6

The Risk Society Revisited

> It is obvious that, in all these instances, the more constantly the persons to be inspected are under the eyes of the persons who should inspect them, the more perfectly will the purpose of the establishment have been attained.
>
> Jeremy Bentham, *Panopticon; or The Inspection House* (1787)

As the number of confirmed cases of COVID-19 in the US soared past 1 million at the beginning of May 2020 – with over 64,000 deaths – President Trump was clear about where the blame should be put. On China. The US administration, after decades of confidence-building between the two nations, began a programme of systematic disengagement with its most important strategic competitor. Business, financial and scientific ties started to be severed. The president instructed his intelligence agencies to continue to search for evidence that the pandemic had its origins in a deliberate or accidental leak from a laboratory in Wuhan. Trump claimed to have already seen such evidence, although none has been published and all reputable authorities have dismissed the idea.

The information war launched by the American government included threats to sue China for reparations, block the entry of Chinese telecommunications companies into US markets, and slow American investment into the country. Diplomatic relations between the world's two superpowers stood at an all-time low. The election of President Biden is unlikely to lead to an immediate reset in the relationship between China and the US. But a return to more traditional and respectful diplomacy between the two nations will provide opportunities for a more constructive conversation about how to learn lessons from the pandemic.

The fallout from the strained relationship between presidents Trump and Xi Jinping cast a shadow over other institutions critical to the control of a pandemic, notably WHO. On 1 May, as he mused on the origins of the virus, President Trump said, 'I think that the World Health Organization should be ashamed of themselves because they're like the public relations agency for China.' He saw WHO as complicit in a cover-up whose consequences had engulfed the world in a global crisis. President Biden will end American hostility towards WHO. He will renew his government's support for agency. And he will stop the blame game about who caused the pandemic. Instead, his focus will be on rescuing his country from further oblivion. With over 20 million cases of COVID-19, 300,000 deaths, and one of the worst mortality rates in the world, the US is facing not only a national tragedy of historic proportions but also international humiliation. Biden is a globalist and a multilateralist. He prefers dialogue to confrontation. And he believes that American engagement with international institutions is beneficial to the US as well as to the rest of the world. But the domestic legacy left to him by President Trump is appallingly demanding. COVID-19 is the biggest peacetime crisis in American history – as it is for much of Latin America and Western Europe.

At such points of political stress, mistrust and suspicion, one might step back to investigate some of the possible reasons for this new moment of uncertainty in international relations and what that uncertainty might mean for our collective future.

In his book *Risk Society*, originally published in 1986, Ulrich Beck argued that the creation of wealth in modern societies was always accompanied by the production of new risks. From the climate crisis to increasing inequality, from cyberattacks to environmental pollution, from biodiversity loss to weapons of mass destruction, we see the truth of Beck's claim in our everyday lives. The emergence of new viruses amid the sprawling cities of rapidly advancing nations is another such risk. Beck sought to prove that our world had become 'reflexive' – many of the problems we face today have been generated by ourselves:

> While all earlier cultures and phases of social development confronted threats in various ways, society today is *confronted by itself* through its dealings with risks. Risks are the reflection of human actions and omissions, the expression of highly developed productive forces. That means that the sources of danger are no longer ignorance but *knowledge*; not a deficient but a perfected mastery over nature; not that which eludes the human grasp but the system of norms and objective constraints established with the industrial epoch.[1]

Beck was especially critical of 'techno-scientific rationality'. He saw modern science as unable to address the 'growing risks and threats from civilization'. He did not blame individual scientists. Instead, he placed responsibility on 'the institutional and methodological approach of the sciences to risks'. He noted that, 'As they are constituted – with their overspecialized division of labor, their concentration on methodology and theory, their externally determined abstinence from practice – the sciences are *entirely incapable* of reacting adequately to civilizational risks.'[2]

These words seem strikingly apposite for understanding what went wrong in the Western response to the SARS-CoV-2 pandemic. The risks we faced, and continue to face, are not only from a new virus. Those risks are also embedded in the systems we have created and put in place to review and adjudicate on the threat of pandemics – the regime of science policymaking.

What constitutes knowledge about a risk, the assumptions we make about that risk, which evidence is ruled in and out of scope for consideration, who is invited to the table to discuss risks, and what type of science is used to shape advice to politicians – these were all weaknesses within the politico-scientific establishments of Washington, London, Paris, Madrid, Rome, Brussels, Delhi, Moscow, Lima and other capitals. Too many governments simply did not consider the research published at the end of January 2020 which set out the magnitude of the threat emerging from Wuhan. They assumed that the most likely danger was a new strain of influenza, not another SARS-like virus. Countries did not reach out to those with first-hand experience of what was taking place in China. And they did not consult experts in intensive-care medicine or respiratory medicine, experts who could have better interpreted the evidence from Wuhan.

As the epidemic unfolded, it became clear that risk was not evenly distributed across societies. In the UK, for example, the Office for National Statistics examined deaths from COVID-19 according to levels of socio-economic deprivation. The mortality rate of those with COVID-19 in the most deprived areas of England was more than double the rate in the least deprived areas – fifty-five deaths per 100,000 population compared with twenty-five deaths per 100,000. Inequality fuelled the accumulating toll of death. COVID-19 has only amplified those long-standing inequalities.

Scientific advice and the political reaction to that advice failed to protect the most vulnerable people in our communities. It is here that presidents and prime ministers should look for answers.

There are also questions to be asked about the international response. WHO moved quickly to declare a PHEIC. Daily press briefings, situation reports and a slew of statistics kept the world informed about the pandemic's evolution. But, looking back with the benefit of hindsight, I think WHO could and should have done more. For example, why didn't the organisation convene nations at an emergency COVID-19 summit immediately after it had declared a PHEIC? By doing so, it could have initiated and led a coordinated global response, pooled evidence and experience, and mobilised and motivated nations to act quickly and decisively. WHO did none of those things. It absented itself from its global leadership role, leaving countries to struggle to respond to COVID-19 alone. The 194 member states of WHO were abandoned and left to pursue 194 separate strategies.

Remarkably, it took until December 2020 before the UN convened a global summit to review the lessons learned from trying to control the pandemic. And even then the gathering failed to produce a significant upgrade in the international response. The UN resolution to call the meeting was passed in November, although the US abstained on the grounds that WHO, their sworn enemy, was to be involved. The conclusion of the meeting was that the sustainable development agenda embodied in seventeen Sustainable Development Goals set in 2016 was now impossible to deliver. The best that could be done was to return to pre-pandemic levels of development by 2030. Global efforts to raise $38 billion for COVID-19 tests, treatments and vaccines managed to garner only $10 billion. No nation took responsibility for global leadership. The absence of the US from its traditional leadership role was palpable. President Trump was absent, sending his widely reviled health and human services secretary, Alex Azar. The UN summit displayed the unravelling of global solidarity that has been the hallmark of the Trump era – indeed, the hallmark of the pandemic. Only the president of the European Council, Charles Michel, proposed the notion of a Global Pandemic Treaty – to enshrine commitments to animal-to-human virus surveillance, acceleration of vaccine research, and health-systems strengthening. But no such treaty was forthcoming. Despite the early roll-out of vaccine programmes, the world ended 2020 in political disarray and disappointment, worsened by the emergence of new and more transmissible coronavirus variants.

*

One of the lessons of the SARS epidemic in 2002–3 was the urgent need for better surveillance of new and emerging infectious diseases. It was thanks to surveillance that up-to-date news of the spread of SARS around the world prevented a truly global pandemic. But serious weaknesses in global surveillance efforts were also identified in the aftermath of that near miss. The systems of surveillance present in 2002–3 were not tuned to look for novel threats. There was little collaboration or coordination between countries. The need for continued and strengthened surveillance was clearly evident if a future pandemic was to be prevented.

The goal of the International Health Regulations (IHR), a set of legally binding rules on all countries, is the control of infectious diseases. The regulations exist to manage new infectious disease risks that human societies create. They were first adopted in 1951 as the International Sanitary Regulations and concerned only six diseases – plague, cholera, typhus, relapsing fever, smallpox and yellow fever. The IHR, as they were subsequently renamed in 1969, required countries to alert WHO to any outbreak of these six diseases.

The toothless IHR manifestly failed to protect global health security during the SARS outbreak of 2002–3. Their revision in 2005 represented a major step forward in international surveillance and security. The regulations now require countries to report any new illness or medical condition that presents (or could present) significant harm to human populations. It is the responsibility of countries to detect, assess and report events that could constitute a PHEIC.

The revised IHR of 2005 expanded the powers of WHO. The agency now had the responsibility to coordinate global surveillance efforts. It and it alone had the power to determine whether a PHEIC existed. And WHO could now advise countries about how best to respond to health emergencies as well as to mobilise financial resources to assist them in doing so. The IHR signalled the pre-eminence of global health over economics, of global governance over national sovereignty.

The IHR also invoked obligations on countries. WHO's member states now had to develop 'core capacities' to deal with major health emergencies. These capacities included expanded laboratory networks, a trained health workforce, surveillance systems, response mechanisms, health service preparedness, risk communication, coordination procedures, and legislation and policymaking – in other words, countries had the responsibility to ensure they had the full ability to detect, assess, report and respond to any new health hazard. The framework of global health security expressed in the IHR was crucial to WHO's pivotal role in calling out COVID-19 as an international health emergency.

But the idea of greater surveillance in society conjures up notions of threats to our privacy and liberty and even, as former UK Supreme Court justice Lord Sumption put it, a 'hysterical slide into a police state'.

Does greater surveillance truly imperil our freedom? In April, the *Financial Times* asked whether the advent of coronavirus apps meant that society was slipping gradually into a surveillance state. Apple and Google were working together to construct a wireless-based contact tracing system to inform someone if they crossed paths with a person who had had COVID-19. Aggressive detection of new cases, contact tracing and quarantine was the public health bulwark necessary to prevent subsequent waves of SARS-CoV-2 infection. Digital surveillance, the *FT* suggested, may become the greatest incursion into privacy our societies have ever seen.

But, so far at least, people seem sanguine. Governments were surprised by the compliance of their usually dissenting and awkward publics during the first wave of the pandemic. They – we – willingly adhered to government demands to stay home under lockdown. The second wave of coronavirus caused more consternation. Resistance to lockdowns grew. The media became more partisan and critical. It's now hard to predict how people will respond to enhanced surveillance in the future. Evidence from past national traumas, such as the Blitz during the Second World War, suggests that people do adapt to danger. Anxiety drives action. Perhaps we will adapt, after all, to greater oversight of our daily lives.

Apple and Google promise that their electronic surveillance

will be voluntary and anonymous. But if surveillance includes cameras on every street corner, the monitoring of credit card transactions, tracking cell phone use, and having to scan QR health codes before entering offices, public buildings and hospitality and entertainment venues, one might not be surprised if the public becomes sceptical about assurances that their privacy will be guaranteed. And if information about your COVID-19 status is necessary for digital surveillance to work, we will come perilously close to introducing 'immunity passports'. An immunity passport sounds a perfectly rational answer to the problem of a pandemic. Such a passport would allow you to go about your usual life while others can be certain of their and your safety.

But immunity passports will also stigmatise those who are not immune, creating a divided society and a class of non-immune individuals who may be seen as a danger to public health. Immunity passports will incentivise efforts to contract infection, with the attendant risk of severe, even fatal, illness. Far better, surely, to accelerate work to distribute a vaccine and offer vaccination certificates instead. A vaccination certificate would shift incentives away from infection and towards immunisation. Enhanced surveillance for emerging infectious agents is essential if future pandemics are to be prevented. Yet there are reasons at least to understand the gravity of the social trend we are likely to see in coming years. Michel Foucault, in his 1975 book *Discipline and Punish*, drew on Jeremy Bentham's idea of the panopticon to identify a growing drift towards what he called a 'disciplinary society'.

In its original conception, the panopticon was an architectural design for a new type of prison.[3] Circular in nature, the building would contain prison cells on its outer curve, while at the centre there would be the prison inspector's lodge. The inspector would be omnipresent, seen without being seen, while prisoners would (and should) always feel themselves under inspection. Bentham saw his panopticon – 'a new mode of obtaining power of mind over mind' – as being applicable to workhouses, poor-houses, factories, 'mad-houses', hospitals, schools and lazarettos (places of quarantine for those with the plague).

Bentham was the first utilitarian. He believed that humankind was governed by pain and pleasure. Utility was that property that tended 'to produce benefit, advantage, pleasure, good, or happiness . . . or . . . to prevent the happening of mischief, pain, evil, or unhappiness to the party whose interest is considered.' The panopticon was an expression of how to weave utilitarianism more deeply into the fabric of society. Total surveillance of the total population is the panopticon taken to its logical extreme. It is the ultimate expression of the disciplinary society. Coronavirus apps might be accelerating us towards Bentham's dream and Foucault's nightmare.

The IHR form a crucial instrument of this modern-day panopticon. They promulgate the idea and practice of omnipresent inspection. They embody a calculus of government oversight that insists on observation with minimal intrusion. They justify permanent surveillance in the name of pleasure over pain. The IHR seem like a clear example of a public good.

But is the apparatus of surveillance also indicative of something more sinister?

Foucault extended his interest in (and concern about) the disciplinary society by introducing the notion of 'biopolitics' – the politics of life. He meant 'the problems posed to governmental practice by phenomena characteristic of a set of living beings forming a population: health, hygiene, birthrate, life expectancy, race ... We know the increasing importance of these problems since the nineteenth century, and the political and economic issues they have raised up to the present.'[4]

Indeed, COVID-19 is about the politics of the body. Foucault argued that the idea of public health emerged with the birth of capitalism in the eighteenth century. The body came to be understood as an instrument of economic production, of labour power, and so became a subject of significant political interest. Medicine and public health were endorsed as tools to enhance these productive forces to ensure that people were fit for work.

The priority given to the body as an important determinant of mercantilist prosperity ran parallel with a further historical turn – the meaning of government. The notion of government began with the narrow objective of retaining jurisdiction over a defined territory. But in the eighteenth century, European governments incorporated the idea of economy into their practice. At that time, economy referred to the family. Advances in statistical measurement brought attention to an entirely new concept for governments to consider – that of population. Governments switched their focus from families to populations as the units on which their political economies depended.

Population became, according to Foucault, 'the ultimate end of government'.

Foucault went on to introduce the idea of 'governmentality' to make sense of this crucial shift from family to population. By governmentality – and the governmentalisation of the state – he meant the exercise of power over populations. We continue to live in this era of governmentality, where individual actions are shaped by power that claims its legitimacy in scientific truth. Public health developed amid these social and political currents. Governments saw the health of populations as the foundation for protecting and augmenting the productive economic forces of the state.

Health became a political problem demanding political control, since 'the problem of sickness among the poor is identified in its economic specificity.' Governments now claimed an interest in controlling and constraining the bodies that made up a population. In Foucault's words: 'Different power apparatuses are called upon to take charge of "bodies", not simply so as to exact blood service from them or levy dues but to help and if necessary constrain them to ensure their own good health.' Why? Because the 'biological traits of a population become relevant factors for economic management.' 'The imperative for health', Foucault wrote, '[is] at once the duty of each and the objective of all.' 'The body is a biopolitical reality; medicine is a biopolitical strategy.' Public health – observation and measurement of sickness, standardisation of knowledge and practice, and the creation of an administrative structure to manage health – became a type of pastoral power with the aim of social and economic development. The growing importance of health to industrial societies led to the valorisation of doctors and the growth of medical science. An alliance formed between medicine and the state – 'a politico-medical hold on a population'.

The practical question was: how does a government regulate, manage and control its people? The answer? 'State control of the biological' and 'the emergence of techniques of power that were essentially centred on the body, on the individual body.' Foucault wrote that 'Biopolitics deals with the population, with the population as a political problem, as a problem that is at once scientific and political, as a biological problem and as power's problem.'[5] And the answer to this 'problem' of the population was 'bioregulation by the State'.

Why is Foucault important for understanding COVID-19? The reasons lie in the sinister way in which attitudes to the pandemic evolved during 2020. It became acceptable to argue that older citizens at risk of COVID-19 were somehow less valuable to society than younger people. It was suggested that young people should be allowed to risk their health in order to protect economies. And governments have enacted extraordinary measures to control and constrain the behaviours of their populations. COVID-19 became a debate about the distribution of power in society – central versus local government, young versus old, rich versus poor, white versus black, health versus the economy.

Those most at risk of COVID-19 are some of the least powerful in our society. Those working in public health do not see themselves as instruments of capitalist states. On the contrary, they view health to be of such intrinsic value that it must be fought for and defended. But we need to be clear-sighted about our alliance with government to address this pandemic. Medicine and public health are being co-opted into a political programme of population control to protect the power of the modern neoliberal state. But the struggle for health should be a struggle for human dignity, liberty and equity. We must also meet our obligation to question power and its effects on truth, on the one hand, and truth and its effects on power, on the other. One important strand of public health is the struggle against subjection.

How do we reconcile the need for greater surveillance to diminish risks of future pandemics – the biopolitical disciplinary society – with a demand to protect the freedoms we have come to take for granted? Does greater surveillance stand in opposition to our right to privacy? Is a disciplinary society, where government increasingly seeks ways to regulate public behaviour, inevitable in an Age of Pandemics? 'We'll keep your love affair secret, say contact tracers', ran one newspaper headline on the same day that one of the leading UK modelling scientists, Professor Neil Ferguson, resigned from SAGE for violating lockdown rules with his married lover.

Somehow we have to find an accommodation. Indeed, an accommodation between liberty and scrutiny is the most important public policy question facing Western societies today.

There are no simple answers. COVID-19 has seen a rebirth of the state. Societies will see the state assume an ever greater role, from reconstructing state-sector economies to expanding social protection, from creating resilient health systems to transforming digital communication, from saving charities to investing even more generously in science. And, as the state expands its reach and remit, at the public's demand, so individual rights risk being curbed in the name of our common human security. We will be transformed into biopolitical citizens.

I don't fear greater state intrusion into our lives – the panopticonisation of society – provided that we insist that this intrusion is guided by some agreed principles, standards and values. There must be a commitment by government, first, to *universality and inalienability* – whatever privacy protections still exist must be afforded to everyone, without exception. Second, to *indivisibility* – our rights are interdependent: it is not for the state to determine which rights it will and will not guarantee. Third, to *equality and non-discrimination* – all human beings are equal in dignity. And, fourth, and in some ways most importantly, to *transparency* – governments must be open about information and their decision-making. Many of the failures in COVID-19 responses had their origin in failures of transparency.

Must we accept and embrace the inevitability of a strengthened surveillance state and disciplinary society after COVID- 19? I do not believe so. Instead, we should be committed to the creation of a vigilant state and society, one in which government and the public work together to identify, monitor and respond to new and emerging risks, while ensuring protections for our most cherished political and social rights.

Eternal vigilance truly is the price of freedom. We cannot afford to repeat the cycle of crisis, harm, action, complacency, neglect and subsequent vulnerability that followed SARS in 2002–3.

*

There is one troubling truth to this discussion of a dawning vigilant state and society. Uncertainty is its foundation.

One surprise as the COVID-19 epidemic unfolded was the immense uncertainty that surrounded what seemed like straightforward questions. Where did this new virus come from (there is evidence that it was circulating before the outbreak in Wuhan)? Why were men more susceptible than women (although not in all countries)? Why were black, Asian and minority ethnic communities at particular risk? Why were those living in care homes so vulnerable? What was a safe distance to maintain between individuals in the street, on public transport or in a queue outside a supermarket? Would wearing a face mask prevent infection or should the wearing of a mask be seen simply as an altruistic act, reducing the risk of someone who might be infected passing the virus on to someone else? Should schools be closed or, since children seemed to be least at risk of severe forms of COVID-19, could they remain open? Should governments shut their borders to prevent the introduction of the virus from other countries or was the volume of its importation so small as to constitute a negligible further risk when there was already ongoing community transmission? After infection, what is the state of an individual's immunity and how long will that immunity last? Was having a BCG vaccination protective against developing COVID-19? Was hydroxychloroquine, a drug widely used to treat malaria, an effective medicine to treat SARS-CoV-2? Does vitamin D protect against severe COVID-19 disease? And were lockdowns even necessary? Could a pandemic be managed by careful and consistent application of assiduous personal hygiene, physical distancing, and intensive testing, contact tracing and isolation?

These questions were asked, but precise and definitive answers were not always immediately available. Instead, advice was given either in the absence of evidence or with only incomplete evidence on which to draw. More questions will inevitably follow. In a small proportion of children, infection seems to cause a delayed-onset illness – paediatric inflammatory multisystem syndrome temporally associated with SARS-CoV-2 (PIMS-TS) – that resembles a rare condition called Kawasaki disease. Why? And what will be the long-term outcomes? Those who are obese seem to be at greater risk of more severe disease. Again, why? What can be done to protect those who are overweight? What is the likelihood of reinfection? Several instances of reinfection have now been reported. Does our immunity to viral infection last only a few months? And what of the phenomenon called Long COVID – symptoms, especially of fatigue and exhaustion, that last several weeks or months after the initial illness?

It proved difficult for clinicians and politicians to manage risk in the face of such uncertainties. These uncertainties only added to the difficulty of planning an exit from lockdown.

Although answers will slowly emerge through further research, the (bio)political management of populations in peacetime, during conflict or at times of crisis will always be predicated on uncertainty. All the more reason, therefore, to have robust protections underpinning government actions in the vigilant state.

*

Two final reflections. Lockdowns around the world have increased some risks and reduced others. The dangers of domestic violence and child maltreatment were sharply increased. The United Nations Population Fund estimated at least 15 million more cases of domestic violence as a result of pandemic restrictions. Repeated lockdowns will only multiply these tragedies. The fund's executive director, Natalia Kanem, called the impact of lockdowns on women 'totally calamitous'. And, in the UK, calls raising concerns about child abuse rose by 20 per cent.

Disruption of health systems and services in low- and middle-income countries is expected to be especially devastating. Timothy Roberton and his colleagues from the Johns Hopkins Bloomberg School of Public Health calculated that the pandemic lockdowns would lead, at the very least, to 253,000 additional deaths of children under five and 12,200 additional maternal deaths across 118 of the poorest countries in the world.[6] The worst case scenario they studied is almost incomprehensible in its horrific proportions – a further 1.2 million child deaths and 56,700 maternal deaths. Alexandra Hogan and a team of scientists at Imperial College London calculated that deaths due to HIV, tuberculosis and malaria could increase over five years by 10 per cent, 20 per cent and 36 per cent, respectively, because of COVID-19 disruptions to timely diagnosis and treatment.[7]

The economic and human costs of lockdowns have been plain for all to see. Scientists at WHO estimated the additional healthcare resources needed to respond to COVID-19 for seventy-three low- and middle-income countries. The total cost was US$52 billion.[8] Outside of the health sector, the impact of COVID-19 has been uniformly devastating. In the UK, the Bank of England predicted the deepest recession for 300 years, together with a sharp rise in unemployment and with no prospect of a quick recovery. While countries such as the US, the UK, Brazil, Spain, France and Italy have indeed suffered economic disaster, not every nation has been so scarred. China became the first G20 economy to bounce back from the pandemic, even before a vaccine became available. In the first quarter of 2020, China's economy shrank by 6.8 per cent, the country's first contraction since 1992. Between July and September, the economy grew by 4.9 per cent. China expects overall growth in 2020 to be positive, at 2 per cent – the only G20 economy expected to achieve this. The International Monetary Fund predicts that the global economy will contract by 4.4 per cent, the sharpest downturn since the Great Depression. China's recovery was a double embarrassment for Western nations. Not only did Europe and the US ignore Chinese warnings about the pandemic, but their overconfidence, even arrogance, has led those same countries to underestimate China's resilience. China's recovery is little short of extraordinary.

Paradoxically, there have also been unexpected benefits from lockdowns. The incidence of road traffic injuries fell. Air quality improved. Greenhouse gas emissions declined. Some estimates put the numbers of deaths averted from these risk reductions in the tens of thousands.

How does a society, even a vigilant society, now navigate between these losses and gains? How do we retain, as far as we can, the benefits we have accrued while eliminating the disadvantages?

Slavoj Žižek, in perhaps the first serious response to COVID-19's implications, predicted the possibility of an 'alternate society' emerging.[9] Although Žižek doesn't believe the pandemic will make us any wiser, he is surely right to argue that 'even horrible events can have unpredictable positive consequences.' He suggests that the responses of governments have made us all communists now. He doesn't mean communist in the Soviet sense. He means communist as an expression of 'new forms of local and global solidarity', 'abandoning market mechanisms' to solve social problems, and avoiding a 'new barbarism'. But his conclusion that COVID-19 has precipitated the 'disintegration of trust' in governments, exposing 'their basic impotence', hardly heralds the moment for a rebirth of humanity.

Ulrich Beck's answer to the dilemmas posed by a risk society was to encourage a more vigorous culture of self-criticism:

Only when medicine opposes medicine, nuclear physics opposes nuclear physics, human genetics opposes human genetics, or information technology opposes information technology can the future that is being brewed up in the test-tube become intelligible and evaluable for the outside world. Enabling self-criticism in all its forms is not some sort of danger, but probably the *only way* that the mistakes that would sooner or later destroy our world can be detected in advance.[10]

The scismologist Lucy Jones put it this way in her book *The Big Ones*: 'Science works only when its practitioners are free to argue opposite sides.' We need to foster better and more informed conversations (and criticisms) about our present and future, about the kinds of people we want to be, about the kind of society we wish to inhabit, and about what we owe to one another.

There is often resistance to this call for greater self-criticism. At the height of the first wave of the pandemic in the UK, when unfavourable comparisons were being drawn between Britain's response to COVID-19 and that of other European countries, Professor Chris Whitty, England's chief medical officer, argued that

We must learn lessons at the right point. But what you don't do, frankly, is do that in the middle of something. We are nowhere near the end of this epidemic. We are through the first phase of this, but there is a very long way to run for every country in the world on this. And I think let's not go charging in on who's won and who's lost at this point . . . Let's do the post-action review, which we absolutely must, at the right moment and we are definitely not at that stage yet.

Now is not the right time to review what went right and what went wrong. That was a common refrain from government scientists and politicians as the pandemic unfolded. And it remains so a year after the pandemic began.

Indeed, those of my colleagues within the medical community who did raise their voices to comment on (and, indeed, to criticise) the UK government's response were frequently 'hammered' by more senior colleagues who urged silence, fearing perhaps retribution in the form of lost government research grant income or future exclusion from powerful and prestigious leadership roles and committees. But those who criticised didn't want 'scalps'; they didn't want to apportion blame to individuals. Instead, they wanted to hold government accountable for its decisions. As one professor of global health, who had spoken out but had been pressured by their own institution to stay silent, wrote to me, 'I just don't understand why academics can't speak freely. Freedom of speech? So many senior people sitting quiet. While thousands die.'

Thankfully their pleas were ignored. Scientific academies, parliamentary committees, think tank reports, and independent commissions all went to work to uncover what had gone wrong. At *The Lancet*, a COVID-19 Commission led by the economist Jeff Sachs brought together teams of international experts to determine the origins of COVID-19 and how to avert future zoonotic pandemics, how to suppress the pandemic and keep the prevalence of the virus as low as possible, the role of frontline health workers in countering political populism, the part played by inequities in our societies, which severely worsened the effects of SARS-CoV-2, how to fill the economic black hole the pandemic has created, how to ensure fair access to new treatments and vaccines, the delivery of a jobs-based green recovery, and how to strengthen global cooperation when faced with a global emergency.

Perhaps we need a different attitude of mind. It is common today to praise the optimist and condemn the pessimist. Who wants to listen to those who spread nothing but gloom? Surely it is better to be an impatient boosterist – to view the world more positively, adopt a can-do approach, be enthusiastic and fearless, believe that our common problems will be solved. We can discover new drugs to disable a virus. We can devise a new vaccine to protect against future infection. We can eliminate the threat of a further pandemic. Maybe.

Yet optimism can also blind us, imbue us with a sense of power and overconfidence, and mask real dangers that need to be embraced, understood, and addressed with humility and care. Human beings are condemned to suffer from optimism bias. We tend to overestimate the likelihood that good things will happen in life.

Benjamin Fondane (1898–1944) was a Romanian Jew who emigrated to France in 1923. He was deported to Auschwitz in 1944 and killed just two weeks before the Soviets arrived the following year to liberate the camp. In his fragmentary writings, Fondane questioned the influence of excessive rationalism as a solution to the predicaments facing humankind:

If the final result of four centuries of humanism and the apotheosis of science has been only a return of the worst horrors . . . the fault lies perhaps with humanism itself, which was too lacking in pessimism, which staked too much on the separate and divine intellect, and neglected more than it ought to have the real man, whom we had treated as an angel only to finally reduce him to a level lower than the beasts.[11]

An appeal for greater pessimism in our dealings with the world may not feel like an inspiring call to avert the next pandemic. But if the scientists and politicians who gave advice and took decisions on our behalf had adopted a little more pessimism in their predictions and policies, the deaths of hundreds of thousands of their fellow citizens around the world would have been avoided.

Pessimism need not kill our hopes for a better future. Hope is a feeling of desire for a particular outcome in our lives. We can protect and, indeed, intensify our hopes through a perspective that does not mask the worst that can happen to us.

*

As we turn to the future, there will be a temptation to say we should be grateful for what we once had before COVID-19. We will be encouraged to be appreciative of the orderliness of our past existence, to be thankful for the harmony of our disharmonies. The status quo ante will be exalted, even glorified. But we must not be tolerant of past conventions. There is a place between normality and utopia, a place towards which it is worth striving. It is up to us now to discover that place. As Herbert Marcuse observed, tolerance 'protects the already established machinery of discrimination'; it is 'an instrument for the continuation of servitude'. If the hope after COVID-19 is for a more humane society – a worthy hope given the devastation this virus has wreaked – we must work hard to cultivate our sensibility for intolerance.

7

Towards the Next Pandemic

The time has come when nations must either accept a hideous death or else care for their bodies as they care for their minds, when governments must embrace the material as well as the rational development of the human race and concern themselves as much with the clothing, diet, gymnastics, and indeed the flesh of the governed, in all its forms, as they do, or are supposed to do, with the people's intelligence.

Michel Chevalier (1832), quoted by François Delaporte,
Disease and Civilization (1986)

COVID-19 brought a divided world together and then divided it still further. The international community failed to unite to defeat the worst consequences of this pandemic. As UN Secretary General António Guterres noted early in the course of the outbreak, COVID-19 unleashed a 'tsunami of hate and xenophobia, scapegoating and scaremongering'. We are still living through a period of unparalleled political, economic, and social anxiety and instability – and will continue to do so for some years to come.

The virus that caused COVID-19 isn't going away. Many countries have already experienced a second wave. For others, a third wave looms. The seasonality of this coronavirus means that it will return again and again and again. The best we can hope for is peaceful coexistence. There will be public inquiries in every country badly scarred by the deaths of so many thousands of citizens. There will certainly be international investigations into the origins, course and outcomes of this pandemic. Long lists of recommendations will be made. Some may even be acted upon. The COVID-19 crisis will give rise to a renewed sense of the centrality of health for the future sustainability of modern society.

Slavoj Žižek is right: disasters can be catalysts for significant and surprising social and political change. Here is what societies must do – what we must hope they do, at least – if they are to prevent the most extreme depredations of the next pandemic.

Within countries, the failed regime of science policymaking will be questioned and overhauled – devising mechanisms to assemble a wider array of specialists to assess and judge risks transparently and more self-critically. Not only will the afferent input to government be improved, but also the efferent response will be optimised to be faster and more decisive. Resilient health systems will be constructed to be better prepared to withstand the shocks of new, suddenly appearing diseases. Health and social care will be integrated into a single healthcare system. A redistribution of esteem will recognise (and reward) key workers. Inequality will rise up the public's list of political priorities. In 2013, the UK's prime minister, Boris Johnson (then mayor of London), argued that 'inequality was essential' for society's success. 'The spirit of envy', he said, was a 'valuable spur to economic activity'. That view will no longer be accepted. Governments will attack inequality with every fibre of their political being. And countries with live-animal markets will begin to close them down.

Internationally, governments will work together to strengthen and reform WHO, the only international agency that can lead and coordinate the global response to a pandemic. The US, under President Biden, will return to the mainstream of multilateral cooperation and will lead new efforts to make the world pandemic proof. To enhance vigilance for new infectious threats, countries will come to view health not merely as a domestic concern but as a foreign policy issue foundational to national security. They will collaborate to ensure that all nations make progress towards the goal of universal health coverage, since individual health security is indispensable for global health security. Countries will cooperate to share data and defeat disinformation. And they will find ways, slowly, to strengthen their own accountability to meet the stringent requirements of the International Health Regulations.

But beyond these important and specific technical advances to enhance human security – advances that will deliver immeasurable co-benefits to society – there will also be momentous changes to the trajectory of humankind. Arundhati Roy has described COVID-19 as 'a portal, a gateway between one world and the next'.[1] What might that other world look like?

COVID-19 will change societies. COVID-19 has revealed the mortal weaknesses of our nation-states. The economic costs – collapsed businesses, rising unemployment, declining growth – will threaten the future of an entire generation. A vigilant state and society will become the new normal. We must embrace it. The threat this pandemic has posed will emphasise the importance of protecting and strengthening the health of civilisations and the natural systems on which they depend – what one might call our planetary health. Our museums are filled with the relics of ancient peoples who once thought their societies were stable and robust. The fragility of our civilisations has been brought into stark relief by COVID-19. The political, economic, social, technological and environmental determinants of a stable and sustainable society will become matters of the utmost political importance. The idea of progress will be redefined – reversal is a permanent possibility. The chief economist of the Bank of England has argued that societies have underestimated the importance of social capital as a counter-cyclical stabilizer.[2] Policymakers will pay more attention to strengthening the network of relationships among people who live and work in their societies.

COVID-19 will change governments. Politicians have understood that a pandemic is a political crisis and not merely a health crisis – pandemics demand leadership at the highest political levels. Presidents and prime ministers have also felt, sometimes through their own illnesses, the responsibility they have been given to protect the lives and livelihoods of their peoples, especially the poorest and most marginalised: relying on markets alone to solve society's problems is not enough. A country's political parties and civil service will recruit more scientists to their ranks. Science literacy will become an increasingly necessary requirement for governing. Governments will take ideas of leadership and cooperation, regionally and globally, more seriously. Efforts to prevent repeated waves of infection will demand historically unrivalled coordination between nations. Governments will learn that acting together, often in synchrony, is a more effective means of defeating a common threat than acting alone. They will understand the importance of public trust for public order. Perhaps politicians will consider redirecting their military budgets towards syndemic prevention – attacking inequality and poor health as well as preventing further waves of infection.

COVID-19 will change publics. Citizens will demand stronger health services and public health systems. Our expectations will rise. We will welcome the rebirth of the state. Health may become an obsession as well as a fear. Concerns about our health and about the risk of further pandemics will trigger debates about the organisation of society. Publics will no longer view disease as a pathology of the body. We will see disease as a pathology of society. People will demand stronger systems of social protection, especially for the most vulnerable. We will rediscover the idea of community. And we will come to accept the risk of infection – and death – as necessary trade-offs to win back precious lost liberties.

COVID-19 will change medicine. The concept of One Health will become a new priority. One Health recognises that the health of humans and the health of animals are intricately connected. Health workers and their institutions will have a larger voice in society. More health workers will be recruited and educated. Public health systems will be strengthened. The well-being of health workers will be held in higher regard. Doctors and medical scientists will sharpen their demands of politicians and ask for greater input into political decision-making. More attention will be paid to the health of key populations – older people living in care homes, black, Asian and minority ethnic communities, migrants and refugees, and those living in circumstances of pervasive deprivation. The way in which care is delivered will be transformed by digital technology, especially in primary care. Investments in medical (and especially in public health) science will be enhanced.

COVID-19 will change science. The pace of research will accelerate, and scientific inquiry will be much more fully integrated into clinical care. COVID-19 proved that science – and randomised controlled trials of new medicines and vaccines in particular – can be done in the middle of pandemic chaos. Research will deliver a new range of technologies to diagnose, treat and prevent COVID-19. Remdesivir received emergency approval by the US Food and Drug Administration. Further antivirals are being studied. Monoclonal antibodies seem especially promising therapies. In October 2020, President Trump received an experimental monoclonal antibody cocktail made by Regeneron Pharmaceuticals. While one cannot prove that his rapid recovery was caused by this new treatment, scientists are sufficiently excited to have put well over one hundred similar antibodies into clinical testing. Antibody cocktails for the prevention and treatment of severe disease will become the norm. Meanwhile, several hundred vaccine candidates have entered preclinical studies. Many are now in late stage clinical trials. The dangers of therapeutic and vaccine nationalism will be severe. A way will be found to ensure fair access to new health technologies. A guiding ethical principle in the science of COVID-19 will be equity – the world's populations must have an equal opportunity to benefit from the products of scientific research. One initiative is already looking hopeful. COVAX is a unique global collaboration to ensure that all participating countries, irrespective of income level, will have equal access to a COVID-19 vaccine. The goal is to have 2 billion doses of vaccine available by the end of 2021 – enough to protect frontline health workers and those in especially vulnerable risk populations. Evidence will assume far greater importance in political decision-making. Transparency around that evidence and its level of certainty will be essential to preserve public trust in science. New fields of knowledge will be created. Zoonotic diseases – caused by a virus, bacterium or parasite jumping from a non-human animal to a human being – will become a supreme scientific concern.

Each of us will have our own observations and interpretations about COVID-19. My hopes are tempered by anxieties.

I worry that our generation of political leaders will be unable to grasp the opportunities presented to them. There is little sign that any leader is currently willing to transcend their sovereign interests. On the contrary, there is ample evidence of an emerging and more ruthless inward-looking nationalism in many countries. There seems to be a view that sovereignty is equivalent to control, and control is our ultimate protection.

This pandemic has shown all too clearly that dominion over one's territory is an illusory security. If sovereignty is the path taken by nation-states, there is no prospect for preventing the worst excesses of a future pandemic.

I worry that many of the issues shaping our future, which were discussed well before COVID-19 struck, will be pushed to one side – poverty, malnutrition, lack of access to education, gender inequality (and inequalities more broadly), the climate emergency, polluted oceans, and war and conflict. You might recognise this list of concerns. They make up some of the Sustainable Development Goals (SDGs), an extraordinary set of political commitments supported by all nations, with a deadline to deliver by 2030. The SDGs are a promise we are making to our children. COVID-19 must not divert us – or not divert us too much – from fulfilling the objective of sustainable human development. We must not pass on the costs of COVID-19 to our next generation.

I worry that one result of COVID-19 will be a repudiation of, and certainly an increased hostility towards, China. The overt racism that COVID-19 brought down on the Chinese people is a mistake as well as a misfortune. China can make an important contribution to solving some of the deepest problems we face as a human community. China's scientific acumen, its ability to innovate, and a desire among its best minds to collaborate – all distinct qualities that I have witnessed grow in Chinese medicine and medical science over two decades – should be welcomed and harnessed for the common global good. Binding China closer to the international community will promote the emergence of common norms among nations. This convergence in values and behaviour was one result of the successful control of SARS in 2002–3. It would be an immense missed opportunity if COVID-19 led to a new phase of dissolution among nations.

I worry that we will lose our capacity to be shocked. Albert Camus, in his 1947 appeal to doctors fighting the plague, wrote, 'You must not, you must never, get used to seeing people die like flies in our streets, the way they are now, and the way they have always done ever since the plague received its name in Athens.'[3] We must retain our ability to be horrified by the incompetence of governments, the corruption of entrusted power and the collusion of elites. And we must be prepared to act on those feelings of horror.

I worry that fear will become a new organising principle of society. That physical distance will evolve as the rule in our relationships. That trust between us will disintegrate. Seats on buses and trains will distance us. Cinemas and theatres will contract their audiences and perhaps their power to move us. Bars and restaurants will put segregation above association. Cultures will wither. Lars Svendsen argues that 'Fear has become a basic characteristic of our entire culture.'[4] What if we create a society that prefers to diminish evil instead of encouraging good? Svendsen points out that fear is closely linked to uncertainty. But, as I have sought to show, uncertainty is foundational to our future. If we allow the fear of uncertainty to engulf us, the costs to life may create an unacceptable deficit for living.

And I worry that we will forget – forget the facts and lessons of COVID-19, just as we forgot the facts and lessons of SARS in 2002–3. Over 1.5 million deaths worldwide surely counts as a significant event in the human story. We should at least consider whether we have an obligation to remember. Of course, families will recall the individual lives lost. But I am asking something more. Do we as a global community have an obligation to remember – not only as an aggregate of individual memories but also as a shared memory that we must act upon? I believe we do, partly because this shared memory is what we owe to those who died and partly because we need to remind ourselves what we must do to prevent this avoidable tragedy from repeating itself. Whether through physical memorials, commemorative ceremonies or communal institutions, the construction of this shared memory matters, since, as Avishai Margalit has pointed out, 'a proper community of memory may help shape a nation.'[5]

COVID-19 has provided us with an opportunity to rethink the ethical basis of our society. The virus took, and continues to take, so many lives. We can't allow ourselves to return to our old worlds as if that fact can somehow be elided. To honour the lives lost we have to live differently. What we face now is not only a political, economic and social predicament of enormous proportions. We also face a moral provocation.

Capitalism has many virtues. But the intense version of capitalism that has emerged over the past forty years, which some critics call neoliberalism, has weakened something essential in the social fabric of our societies. Those weaknesses contributed to the tragic toll of deaths. After COVID-19, it is no longer acceptable to see people as means rather than ends. Once we have resuscitated ourselves from this pandemic, can we seize a moment to redefine our values and our goals together? For we did seem to learn to value one another more during this pandemic. Although isolated, we edged closer together. We took time to ask about each other's health. We relaxed our expectations and became more generous in our praise. We explicitly gave priority to our wellbeing over our wealth.

*

As countries now contemplate the huge task of vaccinating their populations, political leaders might wish to look back to one of the greatest scientific and humanitarian achievements of the twentieth century for guidance. The last case of naturally occurring smallpox was diagnosed in 1977. WHO first made the commitment to eradicate this virus in 1959. The agency intensified its programme in 1967. At that time, 10 to 15 million cases of smallpox were occurring annually in thirty-one endemic countries. The effort required seemed impossible to envision. WHO's smallpox eradication programme was led by D. A. Henderson, a man who can fairly be credited as being the only person responsible for eradicating a disease in the history of humankind. He wrote extensively about the lessons he learned.

Universal political commitment was central to success against smallpox. The role of WHO cannot be overestimated. Although the agency could not compel countries to take smallpox eradication seriously, its moral leadership was crucially important. WHO staff were not merely technical advisors. They became ardent advocates. The agency led the global campaign against smallpox by creating a special targeted programme with a small dedicated staff that emphasised the importance of community-wide disease control. Clear objectives were set. The ultimate goal was eradication. But, along the way, secondary objectives were also set, such as the completeness of reporting individual cases. Quality control of smallpox vaccine was prioritised. The backbone of the effort was decentralised regional and national programme leadership and management. Problem-oriented research underpinned all these actions, solving obstacles as they arose. Finally, certificates of eradication, awarded by independent international commissions, gave confidence to nervous governments that progress was being made. Henderson wrote, 'Extraordinary achievements are possible when countries throughout the world pursue common goals within the structure provided by an international organisation. WHO played this role in the eradication of smallpox.'

The coronavirus we are grappling with today is not smallpox. But the implications for COVID-19 seem clear. First, a global effort to control SARS-CoV-2 demands a global coordinating body – WHO. While the agency's reputation was strengthened by its work on smallpox, the attacks by President Trump have damaged the organisation's international standing. Countries will now have to recommit their support to WHO and its director-general, Tedros Adhanom Ghebreyesus, and boost their investment in the agency. It is WHO that must command the confidence of member states to coordinate the operational response to COVID-19. WHO must mobilise its six regional offices. The US government and its new president have critical parts to play in the renaissance of WHO and resource mobilisation for global COVID-19 control. Second, WHO should create a special time-bound programme for COVID-19 prevention, treatment and control. This programme should set clear, measurable objectives. Eradication will not be one of those objectives. This coronavirus is now too embedded in our communities to be eradicated. But extinguishing community transmission is achievable. Third, countries must prioritise management as much as medicine in their control efforts. Management means a network of trained staff, allocation of sufficient financial resources, investment in logistical capacity, and the development of a realistic operational strategy. Fourth, continued investment into COVID-19 research will be decisive. The first year of the pandemic has revealed the extraordinary contribution of science to our understanding of SARS-CoV-2. Now is not the time to step back from investments in COVID-19 science. And, finally, WHO should create an independent accountability mechanism to monitor country responses and to offer remedies when those responses seem to be insufficient. Henderson's legacy has immediate relevance for today. Every health leader would do well to have a well-thumbed and annotated copy of his account of smallpox eradication by their bedside.[6]

History matters. But the context for the future of global pandemic preparedness is very different to what it was in the 1970s. Two big ideas loom over the next decade. First, the notion of global health security – how we secure countries so as to protect the world. Second, universal health coverage – how we construct health systems to protect our citizens if and when a pandemic strikes. Part of the difficulty is that these two concepts have evolved in parallel, disconnected from each other. In the future, we need to see security as an essential dimension of health and health as a core prerequisite of security.

In a collaboration between academics and policymakers at the foreign affairs think tank Chatham House, Arush Lal and his colleagues have explored what the alignment of global health security with universal health coverage might mean for pandemic preparedness.[7] Global health security means the capacity to prevent, detect and respond to a pandemic threat. The needs of a pandemic-secure country are well understood. They include means to prevent zoonoses, monitor food safety, protect against chemical and radiation exposures, establish effective risk communication, and initiate surveillance at national borders. Detection of new pathogens demands decentralised laboratory capacity, early warning mechanisms and event management capabilities. Emergency responses need people, resources, infrastructure and protocols. Universal health coverage requires a complementary but distinct set of 'building blocks' – a health workforce, health services, information systems, medicines and vaccines, financing and leadership.

COVID-19 exposed the asymmetry between global health security and universal health coverage. The US has the most advanced technologies to ensure its domestic health security. And yet it is the country that most abjectly failed to respond effectively to this pandemic. Why? The reason, at least partly, is because of the country's ludicrously fragmented health system. The UK, by contrast, has a publicly funded universal health-care system that is a model for social protection worldwide. And yet it too failed adequately to prevent, detect and respond to the coronavirus threat.

What does alignment between health security and health-care mean practically? This is the urgent agenda that has to be delivered in the aftermath of the pandemic – in the words of Arush Lal and his colleagues, 'a radically reimagined approach to governance for global health'. First, integration – global health security capabilities must be routinely embedded into comprehensive universal healthcare systems. Second, financing – raising domestic spending on health and moving away from a minimalist focus on 'core capacities'. Third, resilience – the ability to cope with health crises. And, finally, equity – leaving no member of your community behind, by protecting the rights of all, including the most vulnerable, the excluded and the marginalised. There is now no excuse for a repeated future failure. We know how to make our societies secure. The question will be – will political leaders have the courage to invest in the long-term protection of their countries? And will we, the public, have the courage to demand it of them?

*

There is no single final all-encompassing lesson to learn from the COVID-19 pandemic. There is no ultimate meaning to be found in the lives so needlessly lost — except for this thought perhaps.

COVID-19 is not an event. Instead, it has defined the beginning of a new epoch. It took a virus to connect us in life and in death. We understand now, I think, our extraordinary interdependence and unity as a species. Yet our world is organised and ordered by separation, by partition — countries and continents, languages and faiths, political systems and ideological allegiances.

We surely have to use this occasion to resist and to challenge the past mood for estrangement and prejudice. We have to use this time for solidarity, for mutual respect and mutual concern. My health depends on your health. Your health depends on my health. We cannot escape one another. The liberties that we prize so highly depend on the health of all of us. We cannot say that the politics and priorities of my country are of no concern to you. They are, and legitimately so. Just as the politics and priorities of your country are a legitimate interest of mine. Sovereignty is dead.

The post-COVID-19 age will usher in a new era of social and political relations, one in which our liberties will be achieved through new means of collaboration and communication. One can be proud of one's national culture and identity. But COVID-19 also shows the importance we should attach to our global human identity. We are social beings. We are political beings. COVID-19 has taught us that we are mutual beings too.

Epilogue

As I write these concluding words, the final proofs of the research paper describing the safety and efficacy of the Oxford/AstraZeneca COVID-19 vaccine lie on the desk beside me.[1] The article will be published in the next few days. The results reported in the paper open a door to a new year of hope after so much hardship and adversity. The Oxford research describes the results of a phase III randomised trial among 11,636 participants in the UK and Brazil. For those who received two standard doses of the vaccine, the efficacy was 62 per cent, well above the threshold of 50 per cent set by WHO and the US Food and Drug Administration as the minimum level of effectiveness required for vaccine approval. Interestingly, for participants who initially received a low dose of the vaccine followed by a standard dose, vaccine efficacy was 90 per cent, comparable to the efficacy results reported for the BioNTech and Moderna mRNA vaccines. One severe adverse event – a case of transverse myelitis, or inflammation of a segment of the spinal cord – was judged as possibly vaccine related. The Oxford team write that their vaccine 'has an acceptable safety profile and is efficacious against symptomatic COVID-19.' This emotionally neutral scientific prose hides the enormous elation the Oxford data have precipitated. The authors' findings are the first peer-reviewed evidence that induction of immune responses against SARS-CoV-2 provides protection against the disease in humans. They have proven the effectiveness of their virus-vector vaccine in two populations, showing the generalisability of their results between countries. The mRNA vaccines are also stunning scientific success stories. But the Oxford vaccine has the advantage of requiring only fridge temperatures for transportation and storage. One sentence in the manuscript stands out. In small print in the acknowledgements, Sarah Gilbert, Andrew Pollard and others write, 'The authors dedicate this paper to the many healthcare workers who have lost their lives during the pandemic.' The first paper describing the outbreak of COVID-19 in Wuhan and drawing the contours of the pandemic to come was published in *The Lancet* on 24 January. The Oxford paper was published on 8 December – the same day that Margaret Keenan in the UK became the first person to receive the BioNTech/Pfizer vaccine as part of a national immunisation programme. 321 days – a short year.

But the virus is changing. In November 2020, 12 million mink were killed in Denmark. SARS-CoV-2 had jumped from humans back into an animal. In the process of doing so, the genetic code responsible for producing the important spike protein acquired four mutations. This mutant strain of coronavirus, called the delta-FVI spike mutant, was not neutralised as effectively by antibodies from recovered COVID-19 patients when compared with the unmutated virus. The immediate anxiety was that this version of the virus could escape the protection of a successful vaccine. The situation was alarming because the mutant strain had already been passed from mink back into the human population. Delta-FVI had been isolated from twelve people in Denmark. If the efficacy of vaccines was to be assured, the source of the mutant strain had to be eliminated. A cull was the inevitable result.

There are now several worrying examples of mutations developing in SARS-CoV-2. Most mutations lead to virus extinction. But some can confer selective advantages to the virus, enhancing its ability to be transmitted or to cause disease. One mutation that has attracted special interest is called D614G.[2] It is a mutation once again within the genetic sequence that codes for the spike protein. In laboratory studies, D614G increases infectivity. When monitored in human populations, this variant seems to displace its non-variant earlier self. And in animal models of COVID-19, D614G shows enhanced replication in the upper airways and easier transmission from individual to individual. We don't yet know if this particular mutant will come to dominate virus spread. We don't know whether D614G causes more severe disease in human beings. And we don't know whether it can evade the protection of the vaccines that are currently being rolled out in massive national immunisation programmes. But we do know that this version of the virus is associated with higher quantities of pathogen in those infected and that it appears to be associated with a younger age of infection. Another mutant deserving our caution is spike variant N439K.[3] This mutant coronavirus binds more strongly to the receptor ACE2, which enables its entry into the human cell. This variant is also able to escape the effects of antibodies that usually neutralise the virus. The B.1.1.7 lineage, which emerged towards the end of 2020, is a further (although more extreme) example of genetic divergence from the original Wuhan strain.

Not all mutations are bad news. Doctors in Singapore detected a variant of SARS-CoV-2 (one that had part of its genome deleted) that was associated with less severe clinical disease.[4] Those patients who became infected with this mutant coronavirus were less feverish, had less evidence of virus-induced inflammation, and required less supplemental oxygen therapy. Their infection was considerably milder. Evolution can go both ways. Which way SARS-CoV-2 will evolve is currently impossible to predict. Unfortunately, however, large numbers of people are still susceptible to infection. That means the probability of a mutant virus emerging and escaping vaccine protection is non-trivial. (This phenomenon is the reason, for example, why a new type of influenza vaccine is needed every year.) So far, no vaccine variant has replicated sufficiently successfully to present a danger to vaccine programmes. But at this early stage in the pandemic it is too soon to dismiss the possibility of vaccine failure. The difficult truth is that the SARS-CoV-2 virus has the ability to evolve while retaining its ability to cause disease. Monitoring the evolution of this coronavirus will be critically important to ensuring that vaccine programmes are not jeopardised.

Monitoring vaccine confidence will also be necessary. As I work on the Oxford vaccine proofs, news comes through that

35 per cent of the British public say they are unlikely to accept a coronavirus vaccine; 47 per cent worry it will not be effective; 48 per cent are worried about the vaccine's safety; and 55 per cent are concerned about adverse effects. Heidi Larson runs the Vaccine Confidence Project at the London School of Hygiene and Tropical Medicine. In 2020, she completed the world's largest study of trends in vaccine hesitancy.[5] She measured confidence in the importance, safety and effectiveness of vaccines in 149 countries. Confidence in vaccines fell in only five countries between 2018 and 2019 – Afghanistan, Indonesia, Pakistan, the Philippines and South Korea. Larson found that confidence was improving in several European countries, such as France, Italy, Ireland and Finland. Political instability and religious extremism, together with active mobilisation of online misinformation, seem to drive hesitancy. As societies approach a turning point in the pandemic, loss of trust in vaccine programmes is the biggest threat to a future without lockdowns. But, when I look at those countries most severely affected by COVID-19, I don't get the sense that governments fully appreciate the perilous position their vaccine programmes are in. I don't see action to build confidence and trust in a coronavirus vaccine. The longer governments ignore vaccine confidence, the worse the odds of success will be.

*

Why did East Asian countries perform so much better than their counterparts in the West? Gabriel Leung, who was one of the first to identify the threat of a global COVID-19 pandemic, attributes their success to 'sociological imprinting'. The Asian influenza pandemic of 1957, the Hong Kong influenza pandemic of 1968, SARS in 2002–3 and MERS in 2012 showed governments and publics that their region was the origin of major infectious disease outbreaks. People understood the risks. They willingly adhered to government mandates. They also proved that a policy of achieving zero-COVID-19 was effective. In the West, we vacillated. Not only were we too slow, but we didn't seem serious about suppressing the virus in our communities. We fostered debates about the treacherous loss of liberties, the oppressive social impacts of wearing masks, and the intrusion of government into the private lives of citizens. But in China the goal was containment and then suppression. Zero-COVID-19, the cessation of endemic virus transmission, was the objective until a vaccine arrived. It succeeded. A further reason to be hopeful is the rapid improvement in clinical care of patients with COVID-19. Mortality rates have fallen by a third. Clinical guidelines are now available for treating patients. Drugs, such as the steroid dexamethasone, have reduced intensive-care deaths. And a second generation of vaccines is in development.

But could there be another reason why China and surrounding countries have escaped the worst of the pandemic? The disease that follows an infection is not dependent only on the nature of the pathogen. It also depends on the nature of the host – the organism being infected. Us. And, on this question, a remarkable discovery was recently made about COVID-19. The COVID Host Genetics Initiative discovered a region of human DNA on chromosome 3 that was significantly associated with severe COVID-19 disease and hospitalisation. Were some human populations simply more susceptible to infection with this coronavirus? The answer seemed to be, yes.[6] Hugo Zeberg and Svante Pääbo found that this region of chromosome 3 was closely related to a genome sequence in a Neanderthal individual who lived in what is now Croatia around 50,000 years ago.

When Zeberg and Pääbo examined the prevalence of this genetic sequence in the human population today, they discovered that it was rare or absent in East Asians and Africans. Among Europeans and Latin Americans, the sequence was found in 8 per cent and 4 per cent of the population, respectively. The frequency reached 30 per cent among South Asians and 37 per cent among Bangladeshis. This pattern of distribution cannot prove cause and effect, and other structural influences (such as poverty and inequality) are certainly equally if not more important determinants of poor clinical outcomes from COVID-19, but the distribution of this genetic sequence is uncannily similar to the global pattern of mortality seen with COVID-19. An interesting question to ask is why this genetic sequence has been retained in some human populations. Does it, or did it, confer some as yet unknown benefit? Or is it simply a genetic relic of a long-buried era, a relic that might explain why Europe, the Americas and South Asia have been devastated by COVID-19, while China and sub-Saharan Africa have been relatively spared?

*

But there has to be a reckoning. Not retribution or revenge for past mistakes, but an act of accountability. In Bernard-Henri Lévy's *The Virus in the Age of Madness*, the beginnings of a counter-narrative started to emerge.[7] Lévy, a philosopher turned public intellectual of the kind rarely seen in Anglophone countries, argues that there is nothing especially unusual about COVID-19. 'That sort of disaster has always been with us,' he writes. What is different today is how we responded. We reacted with our own epidemic – an epidemic of fear. COVID-19 was 'the victory of the collapsologists', an 'extraordinary global surrender'.

Lévy is especially critical of 'the rise in medical power'. Physicians have been turned into 'supermen and superwomen', endowed with 'extraordinary powers'. Yet the prominence given to doctors has been accompanied by several misconceptions that need to be acknowledged. First, 'there is something a little absurd in the blind confidence we place in them.' Lévy quotes Gaston Bachelard, who made a distinction between the idea of a linear path towards scientific truth and a more erratic journey that involves a series of corrected mistakes. The medical response to COVID-19 was, indeed, a series of errors, corrected after the fact. The notion that this pandemic precipitated an accumulation of scientifically revealed truths is a myth. Second, we initially assumed that doctors and scientists sang with one voice. There was alleged to have been an organised consensus for politicians to draw on at leisure. But as the pandemic proceeded we saw that the science of COVID-19 was, in fact, 'a battlefield', 'a non-stop quarrel'. 'The renowned doctor', Lévy suggested, was 'naked under his white coat'. And, third, we have allowed health to take over our lives and become an obsession. Hygiene has evolved from government guidance to a doctrine for living. 'The will to cure' exposes our preference for some kind of sanitised life, a life free of disease and death – a life that is, of course, impossible to have. And it should also be said that some physicians, those thrust into the media, often next to presidents and prime ministers, seem to have revelled in the spotlight. They have sought to extend our collective pain 'until hell froze over'. They have created 'an incestuous union of the political and medical powers'.

Lévy is right to point out the fractures within the science of COVID-19. But I don't agree with him that doctors and scientists have deliberately sought to amplify their power. It's true that the public doesn't elect experts to lead nations based on their specific expertise. But we have politicians in many countries today who are often illiterate in matters of science. Concepts of risk, epidemiology, and basic principles of public health are not in their usual lexicon. And perhaps they should not be. Pandemics are certain but rare events. Doctors and scientists have been co-opted into government to advise and assist politicians. Far from enjoying or exploiting power, their discomfort has often been palpable.

Closer to the truth, I think, is Mark Honigsbaum. In his book *The Pandemic Century*, Honigsbaum argues that scientific success in understanding a particular infectious threat 'can blind medical researchers' to the 'epidemic lurking just around the corner'.[8] In his study of the history of pandemics, he observes 'the tendency of medical researchers to become prisoners of particular paradigms and theories of disease causation, blinding them to the threats posed by pathogens both known and unknown.' Indeed – and this is certainly true of COVID-19 – 'it would be a mistake to think that simply knowing the identity of a pathogen and the aetiology of a disease is sufficient to bring it under control.' Honigsbaum continues to admonish science and scientists: 'we know better than to trust the pronouncements of experts' who have been 'battered by their repeated failure to predict deadly outbreaks of infectious disease.'

Lévy is also critical of those who embraced the virtues of lockdown (what he calls the idea of our 'delicious confinement') – the rediscovery of nature, clean air, urban silence, even ourselves. He mocks these invocations – 'an embarrassing combination of pious sentiment, bad instincts, and . . . echoes that were regrettable.' Worse, an insult to the poor and precarious. He laments our self-satisfaction, our self-congratulation. What 'deplorable' people we have become. There is no good side to this pandemic. There is no 'historic opportunity'. Instead, there needs to be a political calculation, 'not about our diverting utopias concerning the *world after*, but about the concrete measures to be implemented here and now in the *world during*.' And the prospects seem bleak. Our response to the pandemic may have won our survival, but what kind of life have we achieved? A bare, drained, defeated and terrified life, according to Lévy – 'a life is not a life if it is merely life.'

There are reasons to join with Lévy in his urge to commit to the 'world during'. Perhaps understandably, most attention has been paid to the lives lost during the pandemic. But there is an overlooked consequence of lockdown, one that could scar an entire generation to come. During the first wave of the pandemic, concerns about possible mother-to-child transmission of coronavirus led to soaring rates of Caesarean section. In China, for example, nine out of ten women were sectioned to avoid the risk of viral infection during a normal delivery. But, after birth, the baby was frequently separated from the mother for over a month, again to reduce the risk of infection. The shadow of Zika virus and its deforming effects on the foetus was a powerful argument for taking maximum precautions. But the result has been separation between thousands of mothers and their children at this most important time for human attachment. Rates of breast feeding plummeted. The impact of this imposed severance on a child's development remains unknown. But it is reasonable to believe that the broken bond between parent and child will have had a damaging effect on the infant's motor, cognitive, personal, emotional and social development. The increased incidence of maternal stress and depression during the worst period of the pandemic will also have shaped the early psychosocial environment of the child. A child's development is exquisitely sensitive to this environment. Whether these effects will cause long-lasting harm is uncertain. But the pandemic's influence on our lives could extend for decades to come, not only through 'Long COVID-19' but also through the altered trajectory of child development.

*

The challenge in 2021 and beyond is to scale up vaccine production and distribution. The impression has been given, by scientists as well as politicians, that a vaccine will somehow return our lives to normality by April 2021 (Easter has been invoked as some kind of finishing line). It was understandable that politicians were trying to ignite light to brighten the end of a very dark year. But some difficult facts have to be addressed if public expectations are to be managed successfully.

First, the pandemic is a global event that requires a global solution. To protect us from the threat of COVID-19 means vaccine programmes must have the ambition to immunise everyone in the world. That means we will need over 15 billion doses of the vaccine (most vaccines must be administered twice). The production capacity needed for this scale of vaccination is unprecedented. It will be especially hard for poorer countries across Africa and South-East Asia, where manufacturing capacity is weakest. The goal of vaccination is to achieve herd immunity, which means a level of immunity in society that limits the rate of transmission of the virus. Above the required threshold to achieve herd immunity, and virus transmission will stall. What is that threshold? The level will determine the number of people who will have to be vaccinated to end the pandemic. The fraction of the population, P, that has to be immunised to stop an epidemic can be calculated using a simple equation:

$$P = (1 - 1/R_0)$$

You will recall that R_0 is the basic reproduction number – the average number of secondary cases generated by one primary case of infection in a susceptible population. The R_0 for the initial lineage of SARS-CoV-2 was 2.5. P is therefore $(1 - 1/2.5)$, or 0.6. That figure means that, for a perfect vaccine, one with 100 per cent efficacy, 60 per cent of the world's population will have to be vaccinated to achieve herd immunity – around 4.5 billion people. But the vaccine isn't perfect. The best vaccines currently available are 90 per cent effective. To calculate the proportion of the population that must be vaccinated with an imperfect vaccine, you have to divide P by the vaccine efficacy – 0.6/0.9, or 67 per cent. That increases the number who must be vaccinated to reach herd immunity to 5 billion people. The emergence of new variants of coronavirus with greater trans-missibility (higher values of R_0) will only raise this figure still further. You can see size of the challenge.

Some mathematicians have taken a more optimistic view. By taking account of infection risk at different ages and varying patterns of social activity and mixing, one can recalculate P. When one computes these heterogeneities, the threshold for herd immunity (for the initial virus strain) falls to 43 per cent.[9] Whether the figure for vaccination coverage is 67 per cent or 43 per cent, we should accept it as good news. For a virus such as measles, with an Ro between 12 and 18, the proportion of the population that has to be immunised to reach herd immunity is a staggering 91 to 94 per cent.

But it's even more complicated than I am implying. What if the duration of vaccine protection is short? That might well mean having to vaccinate 5 billion people every year. In any case, with around 130 million new births annually, there will be a constant supply of newly susceptible human beings who will have to be vaccinated to maintain herd immunity. This constant effort to vaccinate to maintain high levels of global population immunity (above 67 per cent) will be critical, since the goal, once herd immunity is achieved, must be to reduce the risk of imported infections triggering epidemics in pockets of the population who remain unprotected.

And vaccine efficacy is only one aspect of the challenge. David Paltiel and his colleagues modelled the possible clinical outcomes of a COVID-19 vaccine.[10] They found that the real-world effectiveness of the vaccine depended on how quickly it could be manufactured, how efficiently it could be distributed, the extent and speed of vaccine coverage, how successful health messaging can be, and how consistently the public continues to adhere to other non-pharmaceutical interventions, such as mask wearing. The bottom line of their analysis was that implementation matters just as much, and maybe more, than vaccine efficacy.

The conclusion I think one has to draw from these calculations is one of modesty and humility. Even with a vaccine that is 90 per cent effective, the world will not have solved COVID-19 by Easter 2021. The uncomfortable truth is that it will take perhaps two to three years before some kind of equilibrium will have been reached, where we have vaccine manufacture at the scale needed, where effective distribution networks and supply chains are in place, and where national vaccination programmes are working efficiently to maintain herd immunity. And, of course, the success of this massive immunisation infrastructure assumes the public will be willing to receive the vaccine.

Epilogue

*

Building and maintaining public trust in the science of COVID-19 is not only important for successful vaccination programmes. It is also necessary for the wider safety of the public through preserving socially protective behaviours. Until stable herd immunity has been achieved nationally and globally, the behavioural changes we have become used to – closer attention to respiratory hygiene, reducing social mixing, physical distancing, masks, limiting mass gatherings – will still have an important part to play in our lives. It would be a mistake to relax our vigilance. It will also be important to build effective testing and tracing systems to identify new infections. Most countries do not yet have effective systems in place where most contacts (over 80 per cent) are identified and results are returned within 24 hours. Even with an effective test and trace system, it will only work if the public adheres to guidance on self-isolation. If this guidance is ignored, as it is in many countries, community transmission of the virus will continue unabated.

A frustrating feature of national responses to the pandemic has been the endless cycling between virus suppression and resurgence. The lockdowns implemented during the first wave, while successful in the short term, were unsustainable in the long term, both socially and economically. In their place have come two instruments – 'circuit-breakers' (planned, limited and strict partial lockdowns) and tiering (regional mandates graded in severity to rates of local virus transmission). Precautionary breaks have been a successful intervention to reduce infections, hospitalisations and deaths.[11] But what these partial lockdowns buy is time to fix other parts of the public health system that can protect communities, especially test, trace and isolate systems. Few governments have been successful at using the time a precautionary break buys to their advantage. The result has been a slow loss of public confidence in such partial lockdowns. Perhaps more feasible is tiering, where different rules on socialising between households, travel restrictions, and closure of retail, hospitality and entertainment venues are applied according to the extent of the epidemic in a particular region. Again, the evidence so far suggests that tiering is successful, especially tiers that apply harsher restrictions, at reducing the spread of infection.[12] But successful tiering also demands political and public support. As seen in several countries, maintaining solidarity depends on the level of trust in government, an especially fragile quality. The emergence of more transmissible coronavirus variants undermines the effectiveness of both partial lockdowns and tiered mandates. With a virus that is evolving to escape our efforts at control, there is little room for compromise.

Trust is a complex phenomenon. There is no simple way to build trust between the public and government authorities. But there are many ways to destroy it, as we have seen from the errors made by governments and scientists during the first phase of the pandemic. If there is the perception that some groups or individuals in society are being favoured, trust will certainly collapse. If the public debate becomes overly politicised and polarised, the public will likely be misled by competing messages. And if public health guidance is shrouded in mystery, again the public are likely to lose confidence in the advice being given. A good example of the importance of trust, transparency and humility in giving advice is mask wearing.

The evidence that mask wearing reduces the chance of viral infection or transmission is real.[13] A summary of the evidence published in June 2020 showed that the risk of infection (SARS, MERS and COVID-19 combined) without a mask might be 17.4 per cent, while with a mask it might be as low as 3.1 per cent. That is a 14.3 per cent absolute risk reduction – a substantial effect. But there is a but – that evidence is of low certainty. In other words, we can't be absolutely sure that masks have this level of impact. The increasing acceptance of the importance of aerosol spread of coronavirus strengthens the argument for mask wearing. Early in the pandemic, scientists believed that coronavirus was transmitted mostly by touching infected surfaces. As time went on, it became clear from sampling air in buildings where there had been known infections that microdroplet spread – aerosols of infection that hang suspended in the atmosphere – was likely an important source of transmission.[14] Nevertheless, the evidence for mask wearing to prevent COVID-19 still remains weak. None of the advice given by government acknowledged this uncertainty. And the guidance to wear masks therefore inevitably caused caustic divisions among commentators. Holger Schünemann, who led the review demonstrating the low certainty effectiveness of masks, argues that, when the public is exposed to a wave of claims, scientists should do more to acknowledge that the evidence on which those claims are made is never perfect.

There is always uncertainty, and, to strengthen and protect public trust, scientists should be more honest and transparent about that uncertainty.

*

Elif Shafak, in her short meditation on living life during the pandemic, *How to Stay Sane in an Age of Division*, recalls seeing signs in London's public parks asking, 'When all this is over, how do you want the world to be different?'[15] This moment was early in the pandemic. Despite the availability of effective vaccines against COVID-19, after a year of this suspended life, individuals, families and communities are suffering from fatigue, despair and misery. Bernard-Henri Lévy seemed to share this more gloomy mood. He was sceptical about the claim that the pandemic has created the conditions for a renewed sense of global togetherness. He is sceptical because these abstract propositions have nothing to do with 'specific lives'. On the contrary, we are actually withdrawing from those who need the greatest help. The UK government proved Lévy's instinct to be correct when it ended its commitment to spending 0.7 per cent of gross national income on overseas development assistance. Aid to the poor was sacrificed to virtue signal a commitment to 'building back better' at home. Lévy argued that the pandemic had led us to retreat behind our borders. 'No longer', he wrote, 'is there any question of a mission in the world or a sense of responsibility for it.' The pandemic had relieved 'us of the burdens of following the vicissitudes of history'.

Mark Honigsbaum also drew discouraging lessons from his studies of pandemics. He wrote that 'in each case the outbreak undermined confidence in the dominant medical and scientific paradigm, highlighting the dangers of over-reliance on particular technologies at the expense of wider ecological insights into disease causation.'

Should we be so despondent? Laura Spinney has written a captivating history of the 1918 influenza pandemic, *Pale Rider: The Spanish Flu of 1918 and How it Changed the World.*[16] She argues that this pandemic, which killed as many as 50 million to 100 million people, left humanity transformed – influenza 'resculpted human populations . . . ushered in universal healthcare . . . accelerated the pace of change . . . [and] helped shape our modern world.' A new era of research into the control of viral diseases was born. Virology and epidemiology were established as respectable disciplines. Attention was drawn to those who seemed most vulnerable – victims of poverty and inequality and those who were malnourished and living in poor housing. Public health was embraced with new political energy. Momentum for socialised medicine grew. 'Health became political.' Indeed, health became a measure of the modernity of a civilisation. Spinney even suggests the pandemic might have brought an end to the First World War. National independence movements were strengthened in India, Egypt and Korea. The pandemic triggered a 'psychological shift' towards irony and absurdity. Art turned to the classical and functional. Positively, and perhaps paradoxically, societies thrived after the influenza pandemic subsided. The 1920s saw a period of flourishing economic growth. Fertility rebounded.

COVID-19 isn't influenza. And its human consequences, so far at least, have not been as severe as they were for influenza in 1918. But we can be sure that COVID-19's effects will be profound and long-lasting. How profound and long-lasting will be up to us. But I will make one tentative prediction.

Western democracies have been struggling for decades to solve a growing number of intricate social and economic predicaments. Plagued by widening inequalities, reduced social mobility, loss of decent jobs, environmental destruction and low growth, democracies have entered a period of crisis. The result has been a reaction by the public against long-established democratic elites. Populist politicians have appealed to public discontent and won elections on platforms of rebellion against past norms of political behaviour and association, from Donald Trump to Boris Johnson, from Andrés Manuel López Obrador to Jair Bolsonaro.

COVID-19 has exposed the catastrophic failures of this populist politics. A politics that draws its strength from dissatisfaction, a politics that moulds its ideas around an array of disaffections, is a politics that leaves hundreds of thousands of its citizens exposed and vulnerable. COVID-19, for all the failures of science policymaking early in the pandemic, has put science in an unexpected and unrivalled position of political power. The pandemic has shifted Western nations away from their democratic traditions towards a new era of technocracy – an alliance between democracy and data. Indeed, the political scientist Anders Esmark has suggested that the opposition between technocracy and populism 'is now the defining political conflict of our era.'[17]

A technocracy is a system of governance in which those with power over our lives are appointed or elected based on their technical or scientific knowledge. Technocracy is therefore more than a rigorous evidence-informed approach to politics and policy. It is the belief that human challenges – from pandemics to the climate emergency, from extreme poverty to gender inequality – have solutions that scientists can discover and act upon. There is no question that the power of politicians and political parties has diminished as the influence of scientists has increased. Our politics is becoming depoliticised. I am not imbuing motive here. As I argued in response to Lévy's critique of medical power, the centrality of science to political decision-making during COVID-19 was not of the scientists' making. But its fact is incontrovertible. Political choices have depended on scientific evidence. Mathematical modelling has shaped precautionary 'circuit-breaks', regional tiering, and strategies for testing and case detection. But the reach of science goes beyond the day-to-day management of the outbreak. Tzvetan Todorov, in his 2006 book *In Defence of the Enlightenment*, asked what kind of intellectual and moral base we should seek to build our communal life in an age where God is dead and our utopias had collapsed. He turned to 'the humanist dimension of the Enlightenment' that was based on several principles. Autonomy – 'giving priority to what individuals decide for themselves'. We should seek 'total freedom to examine, question, criticise, and challenge dogmas and institutions'. Humanism – 'Human beings had to impart meaning to earthly lives.' Universality – 'The demand for equality followed from the principle of universality.' Knowledge was a critical force in this project. And the 'emancipation of knowledge paved the way for the development of science.' But science can all too easily be corrupted into scientism, which then becomes 'a distortion of the Enlightenment, its enemy not its avatar'. Danger comes when political choices are equated with scientific deductions.

The values we have come to embrace – such as who should be valued first when distributing limited supplies of a vaccine – have derived from our knowledge of who is most at risk. In a technocracy, what is good comes only from what is true. In a technocracy, it is assumed that the world is completely knowable. In a technocracy, there is a temptation to rely on scientists to formulate moral norms, even political objectives. The fact that this pandemic will take several years to control means that politics will not return to its pre-COVID-19 state any time soon. Governments will continue to rely on scientists, regulatory agencies and scientific institutions to set the limits of their freedom to govern. Political parties, even political ideologies, will wither. Instead, the next five years will see the birth of a new technopolitics, an implicit social contract between science and government to guide countries through the continuing crisis. Democracy will evolve into biocracy – the growing influence of the biological sciences in society and policymaking.

The outcome of this new covenant between science and

politics isn't yet clear. At one extreme, scientists could remain as servants of power with limited mandates. But those mandates could broaden and scientists or groups of scientists could assume a legitimacy in their role that might be hard for elected politicians to challenge. Still further, scientists could become more firmly embedded within government, with responsibility for political decision-making. Finally, in the most extreme case, scientists could conceivably take over the role of politicians entirely. I don't envisage this last outcome happening easily. But it might be that the pandemic brings new voices into politics, voices from science who, if it had not been for COVID-19, would have remained marginal to political debate. Certainly, I believe that the grip of scientists will tighten around the neck of governments.

Todorov quotes the chemist and politician Antoine Lavoisier – 'the true end of a government should be to increase the joy, happiness, and wellbeing of all individuals.' Will the slide towards technocracy, increasing the power of unelected scientific elites, bring better opportunities to achieve such an end?

Technocratic governments are crisis governments. But scientists are not accountable to the publics they hope to serve. Scientists are no more virtuous than the rest of humanity. Scientists are as corruptible as politicians. Some of the richest and most powerful countries today are living through emergencies and will continue to live through their emergencies for years to come. Technocracy has already won considerable ground during the pandemic. It will continue to do so. Will the newly fashioned technopolitics be able to adapt to the needs of a battered citizenry? One hopes so. But, with a degraded and distrusted political class, the passing of power to science could prove to be a dangerous subversion of what is left of our atrophied democratic values.

Notes

Introduction

1 Elizabeth Derryberry et al., Singing in a silent spring: birds respond to a half-century soundscape reversion during the COVID-19 shutdown, *Science*, 24 September 2020.

2 Fran Robson et al., Coronavirus RNA proofreading: molecular basis and therapeutic targeting, *Cell*, 3 September 2020.

3 Richard Tillett et al., Genomic evidence for reinfection with SARS-CoV-2: a case study, *The Lancet*, 12 October 2020.

4 Merryn Voysey et al., Safety and efficacy of the ChAdOx1 nCoV-19 vaccine (AZD1222) against SARS-CoV-2, *The Lancet*, 8 December 2020.

5 Neil Johnson et al., The online competition between pro- and anti-vaccination views, *Nature*, 13 May 2020.

6 GBD 2019 Risk Factors Collaborators, Global burden of 87 risk factors in 204 countries and territories, 1990–2019, *The Lancet*, 17 October 2020.

7 Emeline Han et al., Lessons learnt from easing COVID-19 restrictions, *The Lancet*, 24 September 2020.

8 Thomas J. Bollyky et al., The relationships between democratic experience, adult health, and cause-specific mortality

in 170 countries between 1980 and 2016, *The Lancet*, 13 March 2019.

9 Daisy Fancourt et al., The Cummings effect: politics, trust, and behaviours during the COVID-19 pandemic, *The Lancet*, 6 August 2020.

Chapter 1 From Wuhan to the World

1 Jasper Fuk-Woo Chan et al., A familial cluster of pneumonia associated with the 2019 novel coronavirus indicating person-to-person transmission, *The Lancet*, 24 January 2020.

2 Chaolin Huang et al., Clinical features of patients infected with 2019 novel coronavirus in Wuhan, China, *The Lancet*, 24 January 2020.

3 Joseph T. Wu et al., Nowcasting and forecasting the potential domestic and international spread of the 2019-nCoV outbreak originating in Wuhan, China, *The Lancet*, 31 January 2020.

4 Adam Kucharski, *The Rules of Contagion: Why Things Spread – and Why They Stop* (London: Profile Books, 2020).

5 Adam J. Kucharski et al., Early dynamics of transmission and control of COVID-19, *Lancet Infectious Diseases*, 11 March 2020.

6 Novel Coronavirus Pneumonia Emergency Response Epidemiology Team, The epidemiological characteristics of an outbreak of 2019 novel coronavirus diseases (COVID-19) – China 2020, *China CDC Weekly*, 2/8 (2020): 113–22.

7 Kiesha Prem et al., The effect of control strategies to reduce social mixing on outcomes of COVID-19 epidemic in Wuhan, China, *Lancet Public Health*, 25 March 2020.

8 Benjamin J. Cowling et al., Impact assessment of non-pharmaceutical interventions against coronavirus disease 2019 and influenza in Hong Kong, *The Lancet*, 17 April 2020.

9 Samantha Brooks et al., The psychological impact of quarantine and how to reduce it, *The Lancet*, 26 February 2020.

10 Jeffrey Sachs et al., Lancet COVID-19 Commission Statement on the occasion of the 75th session of the UN General Assembly, *The Lancet*, 14 September 2020.

Chapter 2   Why Were We Not Prepared?

1 Ian Boyd, We practised for a pandemic, but didn't brace, *Nature*, 30 March 2020, p. 9.

2 Institute of Medicine, *Learning from SARS: Preparing for the Next Disease Outbreak* (Washington, DC: National Academies Press, 2004).

3 Ibid., p. 37.

4 David P. Fidler, *SARS, Governance and the Globalization of Disease* (Basingstoke: Palgrave Macmillan, 2004).

5 Nirmal Kandel et al., Health security capacities in the context of COVID-2019 outbreak, *The Lancet*, 18 March 2020.

Chapter 3   Science: The Paradox of Success and Failure

1 Chaolin Huang et al., Clinical features of patients infected with 2019 novel coronavirus in Wuhan, China, *The Lancet*, 24 January 2020.

2 Jasper Fuk-Woo Chan et al., A familial cluster of pneumonia

associated with the 2019 novel coronavirus indicating person-to-person transmission, *The Lancet*, 24 January 2020.

3 Roujian Lu et al., Genomic characterisation and epidemiology of 2019 novel coronavirus: implications for virus origins and receptor binding, *The Lancet*, 29 January 2020.

4 Joseph T. Wu et al., Nowcasting and forecasting the potential domestic and international spread of the 2019-nCoV outbreak originating in Wuhan, China, *The Lancet*, 31 January 2020.

5 Huijun Chen et al., Clinical characteristics and intrauterine vertical transmission potential of COVID-19 infection in nine pregnant women, *The Lancet*, 12 February 2020.

6 Nanshan Chen et al., Epidemiological and clinical characteristics of 99 cases of 2019 novel coronavirus pneumonia in Wuhan, China, *The Lancet*, 29 January 2020.

7 Xiaobo Yang et al., Clinical course and outcomes of critically ill patients with SARS-CoV-2 pneumonia in Wuhan, China, *Lancet Respiratory Medicine*, 21 February 2020.

8 WHO, *Report of the WHO–China Joint Mission on Coronavirus Disease 2019 (COVID-19), 16–24 February 2020*, www.who.int/docs/default-source/coronaviruse/who-china-joint-mission-on-covid-19-final-report.pdf.

9 Anup Bastola et al., The first 2019 novel coronavirus case in Nepal, *Lancet Infectious Diseases*, 10 February 2020.

10 William Silverstein et al., First imported case of 2019 novel coronavirus in Canada, presenting as mild pneumonia, *The Lancet*, 13 February 2020.

11 Andrea Remuzzi and Giuseppe Remuzzi, COVID-19 and Italy: what next? *The Lancet*, 12 March 2020.

12 Isaac Ghinai et al., First known person-to-person transmission of severe acute respiratory syndrome coronavirus 2 (SARS-CoV-2) in the USA, *The Lancet*, 12 March 2020.

13 Rachael Pung et al., Investigation of three clusters of COVID-19 in Singapore, *The Lancet*, 16 March 2020.

14 Remuzzi and Remuzzi, COVID-19 and Italy: what next?

15 Laurie Garrett, *The Coming Plague: Newly Emerging Diseases in a World out of Balance* (Harmondsworth: Penguin, 1994).

16 Institute of Medicine, *Learning from SARS: Preparing for the Next Disease Outbreak* (Washington, DC: National Academies Press, 2004).

17 Lucy Jones, *The Big Ones: How Natural Disasters Have Shaped Us (and What We can Do about Them)* (London: Icon Books, 2018).

18 Independent Scientific Advisory Group for Emergencies, *COVID-19: What Are the Options for the UK? Recommendations for Government based on an Open and Transparent Examination of the Scientific Evidence*, 12 May 2020, www.independentsage. org/wp-content/uploads/2020/05/The-Independent-SAGE-Report.pdf.

Chapter 4 First Lines of Defence

1 Simiao Chen et al., Fangcang shelter hospitals: a novel concept for responding to public health emergencies, *The Lancet*, 2 April 2020.

2 Sarah Jefferies et al., COVID-19 in New Zealand and the impact of the national response, *Lancet Public Health*, 13 October 2020.

3 Vasilis Kontis et al., Magnitude, demographics, and dynamics of the effect of the first wave of the COVID-19 pandemic on all-cause mortality in 21 industrialised countries, *Nature Medicine*, 14 October 2020.

4 Amitava Banerjee et al., Estimating excess 1-year mortality associated with the COVID-19 pandemic according to underlying conditions and age, *The Lancet*, 12 May 2020.

Chapter 5   The Politics of COVID-19

1 Jacques Ellul, *Propaganda: The Formation of Men's Attitudes* (New York: Alfred A. Knopf, 1965).

2 Didier Fassin, *Life: A Critical User's Manual* (Cambridge: Polity, 2018).

Chapter 6   The Risk Society Revisited

1 Ulrich Beck, *Risk Society: Towards a New Modernity*, trans. Mark Ritter (London: Sage, [1986] 1992), p. 183.

2 Ibid., p. 59.

3 Jeremy Bentham, *The Panopticon Writings* (London: Verso, 1995).

4 Michel Foucault, *The Birth of Biopolitics: Lectures at the Collège de France, 1978–79* (Basingstoke: Palgrave Macmillan, 2008).

5 Michel Foucault, *Society Must Be Defended: Lectures at the Collège de France, 1975–76* (London: Penguin, 2004).

6 Timothy Roberton et al., Early estimates of the indirect effects of the COVID-19 pandemic on maternal and child mortality in

low-income and middle-income countries, *Lancet Global Health*, 12 May 2020.

7 Alexandra Hogan et al., Potential impact of the COVID-19 pandemic on HIV, tuberculosis, and malaria in low-income and middle-income countries, *Lancet Global Health*, 13 July 2020.

8 Tessa Tan-Torres Edejer et al., Projected health-care resource needs for an effective response to COVID-19 in 73 low-income and middle-income countries, *Lancet Global Health*, 9 September 2020.

9 Slavoj Žižek, *Pandemic! COVID-19 Shakes the World* (Cambridge: Polity, 2020).

10 Beck, *Risk Society*, p. 234.

11 Benjamin Fondane, *Existential Monday* (New York: New York Review of Books, 2016).

Chapter 7 Towards the Next Pandemic

1 Arundhati Roy, The pandemic is a portal, *Financial Times*, 3 April 2020.

2 Andy Haldane, Reweaving the social fabric after the crisis, *Financial Times*, 24 April 2020.

3 Albert Camus, How to survive a plague, *Sunday Times*, 10 May 2020.

4 Lars Svendsen, *A Philosophy of Fear*, trans. John Irons (London: Reaktion Books, 2008).

5 Avishai Margalit, *The Ethics of Memory* (Cambridge, MA: Harvard University Press, 2002).

6 D. A. Henderson, *Smallpox: The Death of a Disease* (New York: Prometheus Books, 2009).

7 Arush Lal et al., Fragmented health systems in COVID-19: rectifying the misalignment between global health security and universal health coverage, *The Lancet*, 1 December 2020.

Epilogue

1 Merryn Voysey et al., Safety and efficacy of the ChAdOx1 nCoV-19 vaccine (AZD1222) against SARS-CoV-2, *The Lancet*, 8 December 2020.

2 Erik Volz et al., Evaluating the effects of SARS-CoV-2 spike mutation D614G on transmissibility and pathogenicity, *Cell*, 11 November 2020.

3 Emma C. Thompson et al., The circulating SARS-CoV-2 spike variant N439K maintains fitness while evading antibody-mediated immunity, *bioRxiv*, 5 November 2020.

4 Barnaby E. Young, Effects of a major deletion in the SARS-CoV-2 genome on the severity of infection and the inflammatory response, *The Lancet*, 18 August 2020.

5 Alexandre de Figueiredo et al., Mapping global trends in vaccine confidence and investigating barriers to vaccine uptake, *The Lancet*, 10 September 2020.

6 Hugo Zeberg and Svante Pääbo, The major genetic risk factor for COVID-19 is inherited from Neanderthals, *Nature*, 30 September 2020.

7 Bernard-Henri Lévy, *The Virus in the Age of Madness* (New Haven, CT: Yale University Press, 2020).

8 Mark Honigsbaum, *The Pandemic Century* (Harmondsworth: Penguin, 2020).

9 Tom Britton et al., A mathematical model reveals the influence of population heterogeneity on herd immunity to SARS-CoV-2, *Science*, 23 June 2020.

10 A. David Paltiel et al., Clinical outcomes of a COVID-19 vaccine: implementation over efficacy, *Health Affairs*, January 2021.

11 Matt Keeling et al., Precautionary breaks: planned, limited duration circuit breaks to control the prevalence of COVID-19, *medRxiv*, 14 October 2020.

12 Paul Hunter et al., The effectiveness of the three-tier system of local restrictions for control of COVID-19, *medRxiv*, 24 November 2020.

13 Derek Chu et al., Physical distancing, face masks, and eye protection to prevent person-to-person transmission of SARS-CoV-2, *The Lancet*, 1 June 2020.

14 Yuan Liu et al., Aerodynamic analysis of SARS-CoV-2 in two Wuhan hospitals, *Nature*, 27 April 2020.

15 Elif Shafak, *How to Stay Sane in an Age of Division* (London: Profile Books in association with Wellcome Collection, 2020).

16 Laura Spinney, *Pale Rider: The Spanish Flu of 1918 and How it Changed the World* (London: Vintage, 2018).

17 Anders Esmark, *The New Technocracy* (Bristol: Bristol Uiversity Press, 2020).